Black Men's Health

Yarneccia D. Dyson
Vanessa Robinson-Dooley • Jerry Watson
Editors

Black Men's Health

A Strengths-Based Approach Through
a Social Justice Lens for Helping Professions

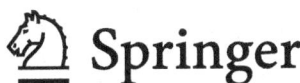 Springer

Editors
Yarneccia D. Dyson
School of Health and Human Sciences
University of North Carolina at Greensboro
Greensboro, NC, USA

Vanessa Robinson-Dooley
School of Social Work
Simmons University
Boston, MA, USA

Jerry Watson
School of Social Work
University of Memphis
Memphis, TN, USA

ISBN 978-3-031-04996-5   ISBN 978-3-031-04994-1   (eBook)
https://doi.org/10.1007/978-3-031-04994-1

This Springer imprint is published by the registered company Springer Nature Switzerland AG
The registered company address is: Gewerbestrasse 11, 6330 Cham, Switzerland

Cover image: Adinkra stamped cloth, Ntonso, Ghana. © Michele Burgess / Alamy Stock Photo

To our fathers, sons, husbands, brothers, nephews, cousins, friends, and all Black men who've experienced or witnessed violence as a result of the ways in which structural racism is embedded within every system in our society…from the education system to the health system and prison system, among the many others. We see you, we love you, we lift you, and we stand with you. Your life, health, strength, and spirit matter to us and we won't stop until there is true justice, equity, inclusion, and access that centers your life, as well.

Foreword

Since their arrival to the United States as enslaved Africans in 1619, Black Americans have toiled under the most strenuous social and economic circumstances to sustain themselves. US residents often identify specific periods or eras in American history that posed unusual individual and collective challenges for themselves and the nation. Yet, the most unimaginable challenges known to American citizens reflect the sustained everyday lives and experiences of Black Americans to date. The nation's denial of Black American humanity validated their subjugation as chattel slaves and disenfranchised citizenship access, which barred their human capital development and the freewill pursuit of life, liberty, and happiness. After enacting targeted US laws which granted Black Americans with freedom, citizenship, equal protection under the law, and suffrage rights, Jim Crow policies and practices were introduced and widely observed across the nation in response to the targeted laws. These racially biased policies and practices levied a crushing defeat on the racial reckoning efforts following the US Civil War and during the Reconstruction period. Institutionalized racism aimed at Black Americans prevailed and the vestiges of centuries' old racial prejudice and bias continue to impact the lives of Black Americans.

The physical and psychological experiences of the duress Black Americans have endured throughout their presence in the United States leave little doubt that their collective health status is enfeebled and fragile. Black men, women and children alike suffer not only because of their shared connection as family and community members but they are also the targets as well as the collateral damage of systemic racist and biased laws, policies, and practices that assault their health and well-being. Black men are uniquely targeted in these well-being assaults on individual, family, and community health and well-being. As male members of an archaic gender-biased American society which largely sanctions male privilege in family instrumental roles and dominion within community leadership spheres, their racial identity denies their privilege and largely invalidates them from enacting expected instrumental and other male leadership roles for which males in American society are held responsible. In short, Black men who are not estranged from their families routinely share commitments to assume individual and family roles and support community well-being for which they have diminished capacity to enact because of racial and gender bias. Not unlike their racial and ethnic male peers, Black men are generally inattentive to their health until poor health impairs some aspect of their life (e.g., sexual relationships, job) or role (e.g., provider, father, spouse) that has higher priority (Griffith et al., 2007). Inability to perform shared and anticipated instrumental, parenting, and social roles affects Black men's health statuses. The Bowman Role Strain and Adaptation Model (2006) was crafted to better understand role strain and adaptation. Across the lifespan, the stressors associated with male gender socialization, economic opportunities, and social marginalization can directly and indirectly contribute to men having poor health behaviors and high mortality.

The COVID-19 pandemic illuminates the social and health disparities that characterize the life course experiences of Black Americans in general, and Black men specifically must navigate in otherwise times of economic growth and tranquility. As the pandemic advanced and ravished American citizens collectively, its devastation uniquely wreaked havoc on Black men's health. Black men are among the nation's most vulnerable citizens as they are usually ineligible from accessing the social safety net because of their male identity. Yet, their multiple exposures to diminished well-being and death are clearly visible as we examine the COVID-19 vulnerabilities and risk factors. Black men routinely experience high rates of housing insecurity and homelessness, two place-based interventions that resulted from adapted and targeted COVID-19 prevention policies. Black men also experience high rates of unemployment, routinely hovering above 40% when discouraged workers are accounted for, but when employed, Black men are more likely to work in 'essential worker' positions such as hospitality, transportation, maintenance, and related work that increased their vulnerability to COVID-19 exposure and infection. Akin to John Henry legend in which the steel-driving man who defeated the steam-powered drill died with a hammer in his hand, COVID-19 replaces the steam-powered machine to which Black men are quite vulnerable. As Johnson and Martin (2020) write, "The John Henry of contemporary social theory is a man striving to get ahead in an unequal society. The effort of confronting that machine, day in and day out, compounded over a lifetime, leads to stress so corrosive that it physically changes bodies, causing Black men to age quicker, become sicker and die younger than nearly any other U.S. demographic group."

In *Black Men's Health: A Strengths-Based Approach for the Helping Professions*, family scholars Yarneccia Dyson, Vanessa Robinson-Dooley and Jerry Watson assemble a collection of empirical health studies focused on Black men in which the contributors employ strengths-based approaches to client engagement and assessment widely associated with social work and other helping professions. The timely arrival of this volume contributes substantively to recent path-breaking empirical health equity scholarship focused on men across racial and ethnic dimensions. The editors distinguish their contribution with a singular focus on Black men's health status, grounding the studies in the state of Black men's health in America and its evolution. They also contribute to advancing the medical, public health, and related scholarship that links Black men's health outcomes and statuses to the social determinants of health and the lived experiences of Black men. By doing so, the editors position the volume to consider the intersection of an economic stressor such as the inability to adjust child support payments and avoid arrearages while incarcerated awaiting a court date as well as being racially profiled by law enforcement pose similar threats to their physical and psychological well-being.

The editors' attentiveness to sharing innovative strategies to engage Black men in research is appreciated. As more empirical studies aimed to improve the health outcomes and statuses of Black men continue to multiply, the voices of Black men in these research endeavors also enhance Black men's personal agency. Their unfiltered perspectives and experiences that shape their understanding of their health statuses are central to the creation of knowledge and skill development in service to the unmet needs of this demographic group. The editors' amplification of the social justice implications of Black men's health signals an overdue departure from the silence and inaction that enshrouds equality and equity engagement for Black men's health. As referenced earlier, the COVID-19 pandemic removed the blinders of segregation and indifference to reveal the social and economic hardships and inequities that the Black community experiences during the nation's best of times. Social protests advocating for racial reckoning across every dimension of well-being for Black Americans remain sustained and garner broad support across the American populace. Black men are highlighted not because they are uniquely affected but as suggested earlier, they are both targeted and collateral damage.

Social and cultural resistance for survival by Black men in America over the many centuries since 1619 is laudable, but like John Henry, at some point, the Black men give way to the collective toll on their human bodies. *Black Men's Health: A Strengths-Based Approach for the Helping Professions* offers a longstanding successful approach to intervention policy research and practice within the helping professions that has rarely been employed with Black men. Kudos to the editors for their successful completion of this volume. We all benefit from their commitment to this important research.

Waldo E. Johnson Jr.   Vice Provost, Office of the Provost,
                                                       Professor and Deputy Dean for Curriculum,
                                                             Crown Family School of Social Work,
                                                                          Policy, and Practice
                                                                    The University of Chicago,
                                                                           Chicago, IL, USA

Reference

Johnson, A., & Martin, N. (2020). *How COVID-19 hollowed out a generation of young black Men.* ProPublica. https://www.propublica.org/article/how-covid-19-hollowed-out-a-generation-of-young-black-men

Preface

There is a need to center the health of Black men in America, as well as ensure that future practitioners are trained to ethically and culturally serve this vulnerable population. Recent surveillance data from the federal government revealed that Black men live 7.1 years less than other racial groups. They also have higher death rates than women for all leading causes of death and experience disproportionately higher death rates in all the leading causes of death.

In addition, 40% of black men die prematurely from cardiovascular disease as compared to 21% of white men. There is also higher incidence and a higher rate of death from oral cancer. These health challenges are preventable and can be avoided through regular contact with a physician. Unfortunately, there are several psychosocial-level factors that dissuade Black men from seeking preventive care.

This textbook provides a strengths-based approach to understanding Black men's health from a variety of angles including social determinants and ranging across topics such as sports, social justice, as well as innovative research methods to engage Black men.

Educators, practitioners, policy makers, and others from various helping-profession fields including social work, nursing, public health, and many others will benefit from the utilization of this text in their classrooms, communities, and organizations, in order to teach and prepare people for working with this community.

The book is broken down into the following parts:

Part I: Racial Disparities and Black Men
Part II: Black Masculinity
Part III: Black Men in Research
Part IV: Social Justice Implications for Black Men's Health

Each chapter includes a glossary of terms and concepts and chapter application/discussion questions.

Greensboro, NC, USA   Yarneccia D. Dyson

Acknowledgments

We, the editors, would like to express our deepest gratitude to everyone that made this edited volume possible. We are especially appreciative of each author for their time, energy, and sacrifice in lending their expertise in writing this book while in the midst of multiple pandemics including the racial unrest and murders of Black men and Black trans men including Ahmaud Arbery, George Floyd, and Tony McDade, among countless others. This book was written with intentionality from an empowerment perspective and covers a range of topics and innovative approaches to supporting Black men and their health and well-being.

Further, we would like to thank Naynette Kennett, Dione King, Ebony Perez, David Rembert, Marco Robinson, Lamont Simmons, and Desiree Steptau-Watson for their valuable feedback and suggestions as we conceptualized and moved forward with producing this critically important work. We would also like to express our gratitude to Waldo E. Johnson for lending his support, encouragement, and excitement for helping us to see this work through.

Finally, we are deeply appreciative of Springer Nature for the opportunity to publish this work centering Black men's health. We are especially grateful to Janet Kim who saw our vision early on and supported amplifying this work and guiding us through the process to ensure that we were able to accomplish our goal in publishing an edited volume that centered Black men and could be used across many different disciplines and settings.

Contents

Part I Racial Disparities and Black Men

1 **Modern Epidemiological Impacts on Black Men's Health:
Using a Social Justice-Oriented Analysis** 3
Raymond Adams

2 **Black Men and Healthy Together: Self-Management
of Chronic Disease and Behavioral Health** 17
Evelina Sterling, Vanessa Robinson-Dooley, Carol Collard, and
Tyler Collette

3 **Positionality and Unpacking Current Perspectives on
Black Male Health Toward Transformative Action** 29
Brian Culp

Part II Black Masculinity

4 **Beyond Moving the Ball in Youth Sports: Making the
Case for Mental Health for Black Youth** 47
Vanessa Robinson-Dooley

5 **The Psychological Colonization of Black Masculinity:
Decolonizing Mainstream Psychology for White Allies
Working in Mental Health with Black Men** 57
Hans Skott-Myhre and Kathleen Skott-Myhre

6 **Black Masculinity Remixed** 69
Troy Harden and John Zeigler

7 **Building a Movement with Black Men: Culture Is the Key** 85
Jerry Watson and Gregory Washington

Part III   Black Men in Research

**8   Asserting Voice: Navigating Service Delivery and
      Community Resources** 101
      Jennifer A. Wade-Berg

**9   "The Talk" Revisited: Expanding the Conversation
      with Black Males in Trauma** 109
      Kara Beckett

10   Innovative Strategies to Engage Black Men in Research 121
      Quienton L. Nichols

Part IV   Social Justice Implications for Black Men's Health

11   Social Justice and Black Men's Health 135
      Shonda K. Lawrence, Jerry Watson, Kristie Lipford, Nathaniel
      Currie, and Malik Cooper

**12   Advocacy, Politics, and the Sporting World's
      Responses to Racial Unrest** 155
      Dewey M. Clayton, Sharon D. Jones-Eversley, and Sharon E. Moore

**13   Social Justice Implications for Black Men's Health:
      Policing Black Bodies** 169
      Michael A. Robinson

Index 181

About the Editors

Yarneccia D. Dyson, PhD, MSW (Lead Editor) is a nationally recognized and award-winning thought leader and higher education strategist with over 18 years' experience in supervisory and leadership roles. Currently, she is an associate professor and department chair of the University of North Carolina Greensboro Department of Social Work and Gerontology Program. She has over 18 years' experience in HIV and STI research, prevention programming, and advocacy efforts. Further, she is passionate about inclusive and equity-centered practices in higher education administration, and her research interests focus on improving the health, access, and well-being of historically oppressed communities, mentoring experiences for Black women and women of color, as well as improving the sexual and reproductive outcomes among women and girls.

Presently, she is the director of the Well-Being, Intersectionality & Sustainability Engagement-Empowerment-Equity Research Lab (The WIS3 Lab) and creator of the *Engag3* Biomedical-Behavioral HIV Prevention Intervention that focuses on decreasing binge drinking while increasing protective sexual health behaviors among Black college students. In addition, this project also explores the sexual decision-making, perception of risk, well-being, and physical health tenets related to Black college students.

Vanessa Robinson-Dooley, PhD, LCSW, CNP received her BA in political science from Spelman College in Atlanta, Georgia. She also holds a master's degree in public administration (MPA) from Drake University and master's (MSW) and PhD in social work from The University of Georgia. Dr. Robinson-Dooley is currently an associate professor at Simmons University in Boston, Massachusetts. She is a licensed clinical social worker in the state of Georgia. Her direct practice (therapist) experience includes individual and family therapy, group work, and assessments. She has also worked in the area of domestic violence, program development, and community organizing. Dr. Robinson-Dooley's research focus includes factors surrounding chronic diseases and behavioral health in African American men, and promoting cultural competency in education and practice. She is Co-PI on an NIH grant with two colleagues from Kennesaw State University, studying self-management of chronic disease and behavioral health for Black men and developing a peer-led curriculum. Dr. Robinson-Dooley teaches courses on "teaching" and is an advocate of UDL (Universal Design for Learning) principles and technology use in the classroom. She has published in multiple journals and presented nationally on various topics related to her teaching and research. She has been invited to speak locally and nationally about her work on intercultural competence, clinical treatment, and managing chronic disease and mental health. She has published in several journal articles and books, and is also the author of a children's book series.

Jerry Watson, PhD, MSW, MBA is an assistant professor and coordinator of the bachelor of social work program at the University of Memphis. Dr. Watson taught sociology and psychology at DePaul University, group work at Aurora University in Chicago, and a variety of social work courses on the bachelor's, master's, and doctoral levels at Jackson State University, Mississippi Valley State University, University of Mississippi, and Rust College. Jerry currently teaches and is the faculty lead at the University of Memphis for social work practice in community and organizations. Dr. Watson is a scholar-activist and generalist practitioner. Jerry has over 50 years of combined experience in teaching, working in a variety of community clinical positions, and leading health and wellness programs and initiatives targeting African American men and boys. Dr. Watson's community experience and scholarship spans broadly across community topics including the following domains with a social justice lens: offender reentry support, affordable housing, community organizing, business development, asset-based community development, cultural activism, youth and family wellness, crime and safety, community violence intervention and prevention, trauma informed care, the "digital divide," race, culture, and poverty.

About the Contributors

Raymond Adams, PhD, MSW, is Associate Professor of Social Work with tenure within the College of Education, Humanities, and Behavioral Sciences at Alabama A&M University in Huntsville, Alabama in the Department of Social Work, Psychology, and Counseling. Raised in Monroe, Louisiana, he earned a Bachelor of Psychology degree from the University of Louisiana at Monroe in Spring 2006, a Master of Social Work degree from Baylor University in the Spring of 2011, and a Doctor of Philosophy in Social Work from Jackson State University in Spring 2019. His research centers on addressing issues of prostate cancer (PrCA) survivorship specifically as it relates to investigating the nexus between mental health, social networks, and spirituality among older, rural African American PrCA survivors. At the 65th CSWE APM in Denver, Colorado, for his publication entitled "Louisiana Black Men at risk for prostate cancer: An Untold Autoethnography" in the Journal of Social Work and Christianity, he was awarded the CRECD (Council on Racial, Ethnic, and Cultural Diversity) Award for PhD Candidates. Moreover, he was awarded the inaugural Frederick Douglass Teaching Scholars Fellowship at West Chester University's Graduate Social Work program in July 2019, where he became the inaugural Frederick Douglass Teaching Fellow teaching a 3-credit hour graduate course for the Graduate Social Work Department. Presently, he is an online MPH graduate student in Jiann-Ping Hsu College of Public Health at Georgia Southern University and serves as a Board Member on the Editorial Board for the Journal of Social Work and Public Health. He provides consultation to community organizations, religious institutions, and educational institutions on the impact of their healthcare policies and culturally-informed interventions on older African and African American men and their families. He is most proud of his role as uncle to Kharion, AJ, and the newest addition, Cairo Ifechi Nmeka, and godfather to Abdoulaye N'diaye.

Kara Beckett, DSW, LCSW, is a Licensed Clinical Social Worker and founder of the Georgia Center for Mental Wellness, LLC, in Atlanta, Georgia. She earned her Bachelor of Science degree in family studies from the University of Maryland, College Park; Master of Social Work degree from Howard University; and Doctor of Social Work degree from Rutgers University. She has more than 20 years of experience in the social work field. As Core Faculty at Walden University, Dr. Beckett advances the field by educating future social work professionals. Her areas of specialization include diversity, mood disorders, and trauma.

Dewey M. Clayton, PhD, is Professor of Political Science at the University of Louisville in Kentucky. His research interests include race, law, and politics; congressional redistricting; voting rights; and social movements (specifically the Civil Rights Movement and the Black Lives Matter Movement). He is the author of the books African Americans and the Politics of Congressional Redistricting (Routledge) and The Presidential Campaign of Barack Obama (Routledge) and numerous scholarly articles. In 2016, he was the recipient of the American Political Science Association Distinguished Teaching Award.

Carol Collard, PhD, LMSW, is an associate professor in the Department of Social Work and Human Services at Kennesaw State University in Kennesaw, Georgia. Her teaching focuses on macro social work as well as foundation courses centered on ethics, social justice and diversity. Dr. Collard's varied research interests include studying the intersection of homelessness and behavioral health disorders, self-efficacy, chronic disease self-management and social entrepreneurship. Professionally, Dr. Collard has been involved in the nonprofit sector serving chronically homeless individuals and families. Currently, Dr. Collard is a co-investigator on a NIH-funded study on chronic disease self-management for low-income African American men.

Tyler Collette, PhD, received his PhD from the University of Texas at San Antonio, where he studied military and cultural health. During his time there, he served as methodologist and statistician for the Latino Health Research Initiative, using his skills to explore health disparities in the area and developing community-based interventions. He has more than 10 years of experience working with diverse communities and exploring psychological phenomena cross-culturally. He is currently a Postdoctoral Fellow in the Office of Research at Kennesaw State University in Kennesaw, Georgia, working on various projects including assisting in developing a self-management curriculum for African American men with multiple chronic health conditions.

Malik Cooper, LSW, is the Director of the Counseling and Social Work Department at KIPP Atlanta Collegiate High School in Georgia. He is also a fourth-year, full-time PhD student and teaching assistant at Whitney M. Young Jr. School of Social Work at Clark Atlanta University in Georgia. Mr. Cooper received his Master of Social Work degree from the University of Pennsylvania. He is an experienced professional in Clinical Counseling and Social Work administration with a demonstrated history of working in the social services and mental healthcare industry. His research interests focus on best practices for African American youth using a trauma-informed care approach.

Brian Culp, EdD, is a Professor and Department Chair in the Wellstar College of Health and Human Services at Kennesaw State University in Kennesaw, Georgia. He has over 20 years of experience assisting communities across the globe in their efforts to eradicate health disparities through a focus on spatiality, justice, and intergenerational physical activity programming. A recipient of several awards for his efforts, Culp has been a Fulbright Scholar in Montreal, Canada.

Nathaniel Currie, DSW, MSW, LCSW, is an assistant professor at Clark Atlanta University, School of Social Work, in Atlanta, Georgia, and adjunct professor in Simmons University, Doctor of Social Work program, in Boston, Massachusetts. He has extensive post-master's practice experience in behavioral health, HIV, LGBTQ issues, men's issues, and community empowerment. He received his DSW from the University of Pennsylvania. He conducts research on trauma, health issues, resiliency, and healing in men. Dr. Currie regularly writes, presents, consults on curriculum, and speaks nationally on the application of Critical Race lens and DEIPAR (diversity, equity, inclusion, intersectionality, power analysis, anti-racist) in social work and other helping professions.

Troy Harden, PhD, LCSW, has over 25 years' experience working in higher education and community settings. His ongoing research interests are in racial equity, community violence, social trauma, and interventions within community and organizational settings. He recently developed and led Northeastern Illinois University's Master of Social Work program in Chicago, and is now Director of the Race and Ethnic Studies Institute (RESI) and faculty in the Department of Sociology at Texas A & M University in College Station. He has worked closely with Communities Partnering for Peace (CP4P), an effort to develop violence interventions for African American and Latino street outreach workers addressing violence in Chicago. As well, he is the lead researcher with the Department of Justice, Bureau of Justice Assistance's Community-based Crime Reduction Grant in Englewood, partnering with the Englewood Public Safety Task Force. He has served as a leadership consultant with multiple institutions on issues of race, gender and poverty, including the City of Chicago's Department of Family Support Services; the Latino Policy Forum; Chicago Public Schools; Fathers, Families, and Healthy Communities; the Pan African Association; the Illinois African American Coalition for Prevention; Burrell Communications and Cook County's Project Brotherhood, a Black men's health clinic. He is also Board President of the Chicago Torture Justice Center, which provides mental health and community services for survivors of police torture by Chicago Police Commander Jon Burge and others impacted by state-sponsored violence. He received an outstanding educator award from Congressman Danny K. Davis in 2017, is a graduate of Loyola University Chicago's Master of Social Work program, and received his doctorate from DePaul University's School of Education.

Sharon D. Jones-Eversley, DrPH, is a tenured associate professor and social epidemiologist at Towson University in Maryland in the Department of Family Studies and Community Development. Her interdisciplinary research expertise is in social epidemiology, family science, and community capacity-building. Her advocacy and research look to better understand intergenerational disease distribution and the continuum of disease-related morbidities that adversely affect Black families and communities. She is concerned about the disproportionate diminished health outcomes, high morbidity and mortality rates, deprivation, injustice, violence, and premature deaths impacting Black families and communities.

Shonda K. Lawrence, PhD, LMSW, MS, is Associate Professor of Social Work and currently serves as Director of the PhD Program and Center for Children and Families at Clark Atlanta University in Atlanta, Georgia. Her research interests include child welfare, the impact of parental incarceration on children and families, African American fatherhood, and data science. She teaches courses in research, data science, social welfare policy, and cultural diversity. Dr. Lawrence has also received foundation, state, and federal funding to conduct research. She has several peerreviewed journal articles, book chapters, and has presented at numerous juried conferences.

Kristie Lipford, PhD, is a medical sociologist specializing in health disparities and clinical research. Currently, she is an assistant professor in the Health Equity and Urban Studies programs at Rhodes College in Memphis, Tennessee. Her research broadly examines health behaviors, urban health services, and the sociocultural determinants of health. Dr. Lipford's past studies have highlighted the role of psychosocial factors and medical mistrust on African American health behaviors. Her most recent work focuses on women's health and the integration of birth doulas in hospital-based maternity care. At Rhodes, she teaches Research Methods in Health Disparities, Social Statistics, and Medical Sociology.

Sharon E. Moore, PhD, is Professor of Social Work at the Raymond A. Kent School of Social Work at the University of Louisville in Kentucky. Part of her current research is devoted to issues related to African American males, caregivers and Black faculty at Predominantly White Institutions (PWIs). She co-edited the text Dilemmas of Black Faculty at Predominantly White Institutions in the United States: Issues in the Post-Multicultural Era (The Edwin Mellen Press). She was awarded the 8th Annual Florence W. Vigilante Award for Scholarly Excellence for the article she coauthored in the Journal of Teaching in Social Work, "The Dehumanization of Black Males by Police: Teaching Social Justice – Black Life Really Does Matter."

Quienton L. Nichols, PhD, is the Associate Dean and Associate Professor of Social Work in the School of Social Work at Fayetteville State University (FSU) in North Carolina. He received his Bachelor and Master of Social Work degrees from the University of Georgia, School of Social Work, in Athens, Georgia, and his PhD in Social Work Administration, Planning and Social Science from Clark Atlanta

University, Whitney M. Young School of Social Work, in Atlanta, Georgia. Dr. Nichols's academic administration includes MSW Director at FSU, Director of the Child Welfare Scholars Program, and Director of Field Education at Kennesaw State University in Kennesaw, Georgia.

Michael A. Robinson, PhD, received his MSSW and PhD from the Raymond A. Kent School of Social Work and Family Science at the University of Louisville. He is currently a professor at the University of Georgia School of Social Work, where he serves as the Director of MSW Admissions. Dr. Robinson also serves as a board member on the Council on Social Work Education (CSWE), where he also serves as the Chair of the Commission for Diversity and Social and Economic Justice. Dr. Robinson has written the 2017 award-winning article, "Black bodies on the ground: Policing disparities in the African American community: A content analysis of newsprint from January 1, 2015 thru December 31, 2015" and also co-authored the 2019 award-winning article, "The dehumanization of Black Males by Police: Teachings in Social Justice—Black Life Really Does Matter." Dr. Robinson is also co-author of the book, *Police Shooting of Unarmed Black Males: Advancing Novel Prevention and Intervention Strategies* (Routledge, 2018). Dr. Robinson continues to publish in the area of police violence against African American men.

Hans Skott-Myhre, PhD, is a professor in the Department of Social Work and Human Services at Kennesaw State University in Kennesaw, Georgia. He is the author of Youth Subcultures as Creative Force: Creating New Spaces for Radical Youth Work (University of Toronto Press), co-author of Habitus of the Hood (The University of Chicago Press), co-editor of With Children and Youth (Wilfrid Laurier University Press) and Youth Work, Early Education and Psychology: Liminal Encounters (Palgrave Macmillan), as well as co-editor of Art as Revolt: Thinking Politics Through Immanent Aesthetics (McGill-Queen's University Press). Most recently he is the author of Post-Capitalist Subjectivity in Literature and Anti-Psychiatry: Reconceptualizing the Self Beyond Capitalism (Routledge). He has published multiple articles, reviews and book chapters.

Kathleen Skott-Myhre, PsyD, is Professor of Psychology at the University of West Georgia. She is the author of Feminist Spirituality under Capitalism: Witches, Fairies and Nomads (Routledge) as well as the co-author of Writing the Family: Women, Auto-ethnography, and Family Work (Sense Publishers). She is co-editor with V. Pacini-Ketchabaw and H.A. Skott-Myhre of Youth Work, Early Education and Psychology: Liminal Encounters (Palgrave Macmillan). She has published multiple articles, reviews and book chapters.

Evelina Sterling, PhD, is a medical sociologist and public health researcher focused primarily on health equity. She has a PhD in sociology from Georgia State University and a master's degree in public health from the Johns Hopkins University. She is also a master certified health education specialist. Currently, she is Associate Professor of Sociology and the Director of Research Development Strategic Initiatives at Kennesaw State University in Kennesaw, Georgia.

Jennifer A. Wade-Berg, PhD, CNP, is Associate Professor of Human Services and Campus Executive Director of the Nonprofit Leadership Alliance Certificate Program. She also serves as Assistant Dean of Student Success in the Wellstar College of Health and Human Services at Kennesaw State University in Kennesaw, Georgia. She received a Bachelor of Arts in Government from Wesleyan University (Connecticut), and master's and doctoral degrees in Public Administration from the University of Georgia. Dr. Wade-Berg has received more than $6 million in private foundation, federal and internal institutional funding. Her teaching emphasis is non-profit management and research interests include cultural competence, sports phi-lanthropy, student success (recruitment, retention and progression to graduation), and nonprofit management.

Gregory Washington, PhD, LCSW, is a professor in the School of Social Work at the University of Memphis, Tennessee. Washington is the Director of the Center for the Advancement of Youth Development, a Program Advisor for the Benjamin L. Hooks Institute for Social Change African American Male Initiative, and the cur-rent Director of the African American Male Academy at the University of Memphis. Dr. Washington works as a community clinical practitioner and has practiced as an individual, family and group therapist in Illinois, Georgia, Arkansas, and Tennessee. His research interests include culturally centered empowerment methods and the risk and protective factors associated with youth development. A major goal of his work is to identify and promote the use of innovative culturally centered group interventions that reduce risk for disparities in behavioral health and incarceration outcomes among young people of color.

John Zeigler, Jr. MSW, is the Director of the Egan Office of Urban Education and Community Partnerships (UECP) at DePaul University in Chicago, Illinois. He pro-vides guidance on UECP's role in advancing an activist scholarship with DePaul faculty and students on engagement with public agencies, community-based orga-nizations and schools. John recognized that the most effective solutions to commu-nity issues should be community-driven. For over 25 years, John has been a researcher, community organizer, and counselor. He's the founder of the African-centered Rites of Passage program called Connextions, which was designed to develop adolescents into conscious community builders. For over 12 years, these students from Chicago's South Side traveled to West Africa, where they went through a rites-of-passage process.

John is senior advisor for the Goldin Institute's Chicago Peace Fellows, where he assists and guides global and local grassroots organizations in building collabora-tive peacebuilding projects. He has been a critical voice in the construction of orga-nizations such as Southwest Youth Services Collaborative; Chicago Survivors; Young Chicago Authors; Fathers, Families and Healthy Communities; and the Rites of Passage program for Chicago CRED (Create Real Economic Destiny).

John received his Master of Social Work from the University of Illinois in Chicago and is adjunct faculty at DePaul University and the Asset-Based Community Development Institute (ABCDI). He is currently finishing his doctorate in education where his research interest is authentic participation of black community-based organizations in the privatized environment of public schools.

Part I
Racial Disparities and Black Men

Chapter 1
Modern Epidemiological Impacts on Black Men's Health: Using a Social Justice-Oriented Analysis

Raymond Adams

Introduction

According to the Pew Research Center Census (2019), African-Americans account for 14% of America's overall population. Of that percentage, 22,458,419 are Black men (PRC, 2019). Despite this fact, a study conducted by Thorpe and Whitfield (2018) found that "Black men exhibit the highest mortality rate and the worse health profile compared to other racial/ethnic groups of men" (p. 185). In general, research has shown that prioritizing interventions, strategies, or initiatives to improve Black men's health nationally and globally has not been fruitful (Griffith et al., 2011a; Griffith, 2016, 2018). Even without considering the intersection of race and gender, evidence supports a lack of investment in general in setting up nationally recognized offices (Nuzzo, 2020) aimed toward achieving equity in men's health, even amid the COVID-19 pandemic (Smith et al., 2020; Pitas & Ehmer, 2020).

Specifically, within the borders of the United States, the wanton disregard for the development and promotion of Black men's health is well-documented (Gilbert et al., 2016; Griffith et al., 2021b; Harley et al., 2020). Griffith (2012) said, "Men's lives and health are rooted in opportunity structures that are shaped by race, ethnicity and other characteristics that have important social, political, economic and cultural meaning" (p. 106). This book chapter aims to display from a non-deficit frame how Black men's survival too often is contingent not only on mitigating unfavorable social determinants of health within their social ecologies but also on installing interlocking mutually beneficial systems. Divulging the epidemiological effects of how such determinants affect their overall well-being can inform how we, as change agents (e.g., social workers), implement modalities geared toward improving their lives.

R. Adams (✉)
Department of Social Work, Counseling & Psychology, Alabama A&M University, Huntsville, AL, USA
e-mail: raymond.adams@aamu.edu

© The Author(s), under exclusive license to Springer Nature Switzerland AG 2022
Y. D. Dyson et al. (eds.), *Black Men's Health*, https://doi.org/10.1007/978-3-031-04994-1_1

However, before discussing more relevant statistical factors, it becomes essential to situate this male ethnic group's health inequities within a sound theoretical orientation. In the section that follows, I will supply a brief overview of social capital theory, which espouses that "Social capital can also be viewed as social resources embedded from individuals' social relationships in their local communities and/or family systems where they have shared norms, values, and common memberships" (Zhang & Lu, 2019, p. 2). This will allow the readers to understand the relationships between individuals, systems, and various organizations particularly among this male ethnic group (e.g., Black men).

Social Capital Analysis of Health

Different scholars' (Bourdieu, 1986; Coleman, 1988, 1990; Lin, 1999; Putnam, 1993, 1995) conceptualization of social capital theory has led to methodological and definitional unclarity. However, for this book chapter, the author will define the theory "as features of social organization, such as trust, norms, and networks that can improve the efficiency of society by facilitating coordinated action" (Zhang & Lu, 2019, p. 2). With this in mind, among Black men, the linkage between social capital and health directly correlates to positive outcomes and behaviors (Dean et al., 2015). Specifically, a recent study conducted by Cain et al. (2017) discovered that "there is a long history of research showing that higher social capital improves health, above and beyond individual-level characteristics" (p. 2). It is necessary to discuss social scientists' underutilization of the social cohesiveness of African-American communities. Too often, social scientists ignore the influences of social capital and social networks inherent within African diasporic communities.

The literature denotes five concepts of social capital—(1) bonding, (2) bridging, (3) cognitive, (4) structural, and (5) linking—that, if synchronized, can help establish positive social capital and access to new social networks (Aldrich & Meyer, 2015; Boeri et al., 2016). To fully understand *social capital*, it is necessary to define each of the five components. *Bonding* refers to emotionally bonded groups such as friends and family. For instance, a study conducted by Robinson et al. (2018) has shown that the bonding experiences Black males engage in within the social institution of the Black church have positive effects on their overall well-being and mental health. Renowned Black scholar Derrick Brooms (2020) underscores that "An important aspect of Black men's engagement is their bonding relationships with each other and identity" (p. 2). As we pivot to the concept of *bridging*, which Hussen et al. (2018) refer to as "resources derived from cross-identity connections" (p. 52), it becomes essential to understand that bridging refers to weak affiliations among heterogeneous groups such as siblings or church members (Amoah et al., 2018; Boeri et al., 2016).

As it relates to Black men's health, as mentioned earlier, there has been a weak historical relationship between governmental health institutions and us (Griffith et al., 2011b). In that same vein, Griffith et al. (2021a) states that, "Given this history, it would be illogical and irrational not to approach providers and healthcare entities with some level of skepticism" (p. 1). Therefore, it become incumbent upon workers who supply healthcare-related services to understand how this "healthy cultural paranoia" Griffith et al. (2021a, p. 1) can inform their respective healthcare practices when in engaging Black men. This healthy skepticism regarding health-care systems routinely discussed with trusted individuals within our social networks (e.g., churches, social groups, friends, family, etc.).

A study by Hussen et al. (2018) suggests that "Both bonding and bridging capital can be used to elicit new and useful resilience resources, such as informational support, instrumental support, emotional support; and they can also be used to build collective efficacy (an asset)" (p. 52). Another critical aspect of social capital is what Verduin et al. (2014) describes as, "*Structural* and *cognitive* social capital, respectively, can be characterized as what people 'do' and what people 'feel' in terms of social relations" (p. 2). These two concepts of social capital are typically defined separately in the larger body of literature (Nyqvist et al., 2014). However, in this instance, as the author, I purposefully combine the two concepts to explicate Black men's psychosocial connectivity within their social ecologies. For example, Nguyen et al. (2019a) presented significant analysis and discussion on the subject of social isolation among African-Americans and its associative impact on their psychiatric health.

Black scholars consistently point toward gaps in knowledge regarding Black men's psychological well-being, as well as why the broader literature warrants more in-depth investigative approaches regarding this issue (Allen et al., 2019; Johnson-Lawrence et al., 2013; Lincoln et al., 2011; Watkins et al., 2010, 2011, 2015). Despite this, little progress has been made in the investigation of setting up Boeri et al. (2016)'s concept of *linking social capital*, which "refers to connections that cross social class divisions" (p. 2). Griffith et al. (2021b)'s research "highlight the need to consider how the context of health behavior and the meaning ascribed to certain behaviors are gendered, not only from a man's perspective, but also how his social networks, behavioral context, and the dynamic sociopolitical climate may consider gendered ideals in ways that shape behavior" (p. 1).

For instance, Santee et al. (2018) suggest that "Cancer survivors connected to a diverse range of individuals may have increased rates of survival, whereas those who are isolated may have increased risk of functional decline" (p. 11). Recent scholarship by Adams (2019) and Adams and Johnson Jr., (2021), exploration of faith and prostate cancer survivorship among African-American PrCA cancer survivors, supports the preceding statement. Nevertheless, this section has attempted to provide a brief summary of the literature relating to how the five components of social capital theory can potentially assist social work and public health practitioners in moving toward a more culturally situated perception and interpretation of Black men's health within the context it occurs.

In the next section that follows, I briefly argue that the concept of "John Henryism" (Bennett et al., 2004; James, 1994), a perspective that Lopes et al. (2018) defined as "A strong behavioral or personality predisposition to engage in high-effort coping with difficult socio-environmental stressors" (p. 539), must be interwoven into how to best conceptualize Black men's health given how we are disproportionately impacted by social, psychological, political, and environmental stressors. This conceptualization, in particular, must be firmly etched into the minds of social work and public health practitioners as it adequately demonstrates how some Black men feel they must persevere regardless of the imposed barriers within their situated social ecologies. Suffer no delusions as the readers of this chapter; Black men's historical and modern-day issues are due primarily to US society's unwillingness to engage in transformative and emancipatory practices aimed at our liberation and preservation.

Literature Review

As Black scholars try to rebound after four years of disinformation and "fake news" under the Trump administration, it becomes imperative we hold firm to our commitment to showing the true meaning of why *#BlackLivesMatter* to those of us committed to our survival. It would be useful at this stage to consider what the literature reveals to be pertinent social determinants of health among Black men (Xanthos et al., 2010).

Social determinants of health (SDoH) refer to "conditions in the places where people live, learn, work, and play that affect a wide range of health risks and outcomes" (Turner-Musa et al., 2020, p. 2). Having now defined what is meant by SDoH, I will now move on to discuss a few SDoH, which negatively affect Black men's overall health within the United States. On the question of "prisoner reentry industry (PRI)," Ortiz and Jackey (2019) posited "it is an intentional form of structural violence perpetuated by the state to ensure the continued oppression of the most marginalized groups in our society" (p. 484). Notable scholars such as Smith and Hattery (2010) continue to argue "the linkages between the mass incarceration of African American men by the Prison Industrial Complex (PIC) and the consequent bleeding of capital—specifically financial, human, social and political from the men themselves, their families, and the African American community at large" (p. 388). Recently, Williams et al. (2019) critical ethnography discovered that "Black males are over-represented in state and federal prisons throughout the United States" (p. 438).

This overrepresentation has far-reaching implications on their overall health particularly among incarcerated older adults (Jang & Canada, 2014). Specifically, another study by Williams et al. (2020) found that formerly incarcerated Black males' dietary habits became compromised due to poor food quality during their tenure in prison. It has been conclusively shown that "Critical gerontological knowledge and skills needed in prison healthcare include awareness regarding the unusual clinical presentations of COVID-19 among older adults, deconditioning among older adults due to immobility, challenges in prognostication, and advance care planning with older adults" (Prost et al., 2021, p. 3).

To further examine the role of COVID-19 infections in US jails and prisons among African-Americans, Franco-Parede et al. (2020, 2021) carried out a series of studies to extrapolate prison healthcare disproportionality among this targeted male population. It has been studied by leading researchers that there is a low participation rate among Black detained and incarcerated persons to even take the COVID-19 vaccination (Stern et al., 2021). The study mentioned above regarding vaccine hesitancy among detained and incarcerated persons serves as an excellent example of why more empirical investigations must explore more detailed nuances of how continuously Black men are disadvantaged by a system not built for their preservation.

In the literature, the COVID-19 global pandemic has shown its ability to uncover how overall generational poverty impacts African-Americans and how it will prevent them from establishing generation wealth or improved health outcomes (Snowden & Graaf, 2021). This discovery should lead to new understandings of the intersection of prison healthcare practices, deficient infrastructures, and infectious diseases that can affect Black men's health. Having argued the role of the prison industrial complex within the lives of Black men's health, one must be open to discussing how policing contributes to their Black men's health destabilization (Gilbert et al., 2016). Let us now turn to discuss Bowleg et al. (2020)'s research which seeks "To examine negative police encounters and police avoidance as mediators of incarceration history and depressive symptoms among US Black men and to assess the role of unemployment as a moderator of these associations" (p. 1). In the next section, I will present the principal findings of the current data on the intersection of policing and Black men and its profound impact on their overall physical and mental health.

It is widely acknowledged that "hyper-policing" (Bowleg et al., 2020) defined as "an aggressive form of policing characterized by intensive and extensive police surveillance, the "noticing" of crime in racial/ethnic minority neighborhoods, and the designation of entire neighborhoods and residents as potential or actual criminals (p. 1) has systemically and historically permeated Black communities (Williams, 2017, 2019). Situating this aggressive form of policing as an SDoH became vital in the wake of the highly televised and politicized state-sanctioned police murder of George Floyd. As said previously, as a Black scholar, I must be about the business of naming and giving meaning to why #BlackLivesMatter for us who continue to exist on the margins of society (e.g., Black men). Before I begin expounding on statistical data to support this justification, it is incumbent I state my socially located privilege. As a Black male academician, I wholeheartedly recognize I have no guaranteed exemption from "hyper-policing" (Bowleg et al., 2020) simply due to my proximity and presence on the modern-day slave plantation (e.g., college and universities) where I work as a tenured faculty member.

However, my intersectional identities allow me the privilege of espousing my proximity while simultaneously discussing its harmful effects on members within my own male-ethnic group. Therefore, desegregating my race and gender from this analysis as a form of objectivity is impossible; asking me to do so would suggest you stand on the side of oppression instead of justice. With that said, the academic literature on policing practices among and between Black men and boys has revealed the emergence of a not only a modern but also relevant sociohistorical racialized trend (Brooks et al., 2016; Brooms & Perry, 2016; Brooms & Clark, 2020; Campbell & Valera, 2020; Jackson et al., 2020; Johnson et al., 2019; Staggers-Hakim, 2016; Moore et al., 2016; Obasogie & Newman, 2017).

Obviously, the movement toward purging these racist degenerates from the US police forces has met resistance at almost every level of government (Hutto & Green, 2016; Mrozla et al., 2021). Many individuals who conduct research on police abolition and defunding (e.g., Jacobs et al., 2021; Kim, 2020; McGee, 2021; Preston, 2021; Richie & Martensen, 2020) have offered recommendations and examined ways to resisting carcerality within the US landscape. Such proposals are based on the direct linkage between American policing and Black health (Alang et al., 2017). Even so, members of this racial group have formulated the conclusion that embedding these kinds of racist officers in law enforcement is pivotal to the preservation of the US white supremacist injustice system. Historically, the maintenance of this ideology comes from the intergenerational traumas incurred through slave patrols to Black Codes, to Civil Rights era terrorism, and the present-day mass incarceration of Black and Brown bodies (Durr, 2015; Hill, 2020; Williams, 2019).

If we frame this form of psychosocial oppression as experienced by Black individuals amid the COVID-19 pandemic (Gonzales et al., 2021), one can learn the true depth and breadth of its impact on their everyday lives. Given this evidence, it becomes incumbent that social work and public health practitioners do not view such intersectional vulnerabilities as situational occurrences. More research is needed to develop a deeper understanding of the relationship between policing and Black male survivorship; however, instead of continuing dwelling on the negative SDoH, it is important to accentuate elements of our intersectional identities that buffer such atrocities. The following section will discuss two SDoH (i.e., faith and spirituality) provided through church-based supports (Nguyen et al., 2019a).

Faith and Spirituality

My anti-integrationist spiritual ethos will forever be set ablaze by every word uttered by the belated Honorable Brother El-Hajj Malik El-Shabazz, known historically as Malcolm X. His gifted lexicon to this day gives me profound insight into both past and modern perils of being a Black man in America. Regardless of the context or situation, he proselytized unabashedly and unapologetically about our trials and tribulations specifically as Black men. Case in point, studies conducted by Graham et al. (2017) support that "Boys and men of color are exposed to traumatic experiences at significantly higher rates than are other demographic groups" (p. 1). Another study found that, "Urban black men from disadvantaged neighborhoods have life experiences such as exposure to racism, poverty, and other traumas, and these cumulative exposures add to the psychological burden that likely contributes to the severity of post-injury depression and PTSD symptoms" (Richmond et al.,

2019, p. 837). Social work scholars have recently begun researching an understudied phenomenon about our constant exposure to community-based violence via social media (Motley et al., 2020). Despite these compounding traumatic exposures, our conceptualization of "faith" (Adams & Johnson Jr., 2021) has continued to serve as a meaningful form of mediation toward our intersectional oppressions. Central to the theory of critical race is the tenet of counter-storytelling. This tenet supports the usage of various literary sources to expound upon the lived experiences of minoritized individuals (Solórzano et al., 2000).

Significance to Social Work and Public Health

Research continues to struggle to authentically contextualize how the psychosocial functioning of African-American men is affected by the everyday challenges presented by culture, economics, and geographical locations (i.e., rural areas). Therefore, this book chapter looks to advance the field of social work and public health by qualitatively exploring how this male-ethnic group interprets and gives meaning to their survivorship within their social ecologies. The findings and conclusions may potentially inform culturally-relevant interventions related to psychosocial functioning and affect how processes are developed. Furthermore, "trauma in childhood can affect health at each life stage, is cumulative, and can detrimentally impact mental and physical health and social advantage of subsequent generations" (Goldstein et al., 2020, p. 187), which further justifies the implementation of more gendered and culturally nuanced based interventions among these Black men and boys to evoke healthcare changes.

Summary
This book chapter is presented in two chapters. In this chapter provides an overview of selected social determinants of health for Black men. Specifically, the author provides information on the prevalence, incidences, risk factors, survivorship, prognosis, interventions, and treatment. Chapter 2 examines the body of literature significant to the study by expounding on factors relevant to the psychosocial functioning of this specific male ethnic group. Furthermore, the author expands on the prevalence of these determinants through primarily through the theoretical frame of social capital theory to extrapolate the intersecting vulnerabilities' that they face systemically. Finally, the Discussion questions and Chapter Exercises discuss the onus to which social work and public health practitioners can reflect on divulging ways to solidify their commitment to the social uplift of men within the African diaspora.

Discussion Questions

1. How do conversations about the intersections of race, white privilege, social oppression, etc. among Black men show up in social work and public health programs?

2. Do administrators use specific anti-racism-focused assignments or co-conspirator frameworks when covering these issues in field seminars and practice-oriented courses?
3. How can you boost the ability of your key administrators (e.g., Program Directors, Deans, and Department Chairs) to be able to implement strategic conversations about the intersectional vulnerabilities among Black men with their students given what they will meet outside the academic setting pre- and postgraduates?

Exercises
1. As a group, students will research at least three social determinants of health that disproportionately affect Black men and construct an infographic sketch that appropriately disaggregates each determinant of health's impact on Black men's lives.
2. Each student in a group of three will develop a gender-based psychosocial group that speaks to addressing a specific social determinant of health (e.g., depression, heart diseases, poverty) as experienced by Black men in rural areas.
3. Each student will construct a policy brief regarding the role of Black Churches in health promotion activities among Black men.

Glossary of Terms and Concepts
Described in this section are the terms presented throughout these chapters. The sole purpose of these definitions is to provide transparency in how the author utilizes them in this book chapter.

African-American and Black men: Based on the heterogeneity of the male-ethnic group within this study, these labels will be interchangeably utilized (Agyemang et al., 2005).
Counter-storytelling: This is a critical race theory (CRT) tenet which allow various mediums of narration (e.g., storytelling, biographies scenarios, parables) to elucidate and disrupt white dominant ideological frames of knowing, experiences, and research (Parker, 2015; Solórzano et al., 2000).
Spirituality: In this present chapter, this term is defined and contextualized as the embodiment of socio-historical tenets of Judeo-Christian dogma, beliefs, and values as understood by members of the African diaspora (Cone, 1986; Harvey, 2013; Taylor & Chatters, 2010; Taylor et al., 2014).
Social Networks: Throughout this chapter, this term is used to refer to informal systems as well as formal systems of social supports among African-Americans (Taylor et al., 2017; Nguyen et al., 2016, 2019a, b).
Rural and Rurality: According to a definition provided by the US Census (2016), rural "Is defined as all population, housing, and territory not included within an urbanized area or urban cluster" (p. 3); as such, this study has chosen to utilize it interchangeably through this chapter.
Mental Illness: The definitional clarity between the two term's mental health (Galderisi et al., 2015) and mental illness (Sickel et al., 2019) within the broader literature is often ambiguous if not synonymous. For clarity, in this chapter, it's

seen as the existence of one or more emotional disturbances as defined by the *Diagnostic and Statistical Manual of Mental Disorders, Fifth Edition* (DSM-5) (Ahonen et al. 2019).

Mental Health: This is the term that denotes "a state of well-being in which the individual realizes his or her own abilities, can cope with the normal stresses of life, can work productively and fruitfully, and is able to make a contribution to his or her community" (Westerhof & Keyes, 2010, p. 111).

Quality of Life (QOL): This is the term that denotes physical, psychological, social, and spiritual well-being can be perceived, experienced, and interpreted differently by an individual (Dickey & Ogunsanya, 2018).

Social determinants of health (SDoH) refer to "conditions in the places where people live, learn, work, and play that affect a wide range of health risks and outcomes" (Turner-Musa et al., 2020, p. 2).

References

Adams, R. D. (2019). Louisiana Black Men at risk for prostate cancer: An Untold Autoethnography. *Journal of Social Work and Christianity, 46*(1), 49–59.

Adams, R. D., & Johnson, W. E., Jr. (2021). Faith as a mechanism for health promotion among Rural African American Prostate Cancer Survivors: A qualitative examination. *International Journal of Environmental Research and Public Health, 18*(6), 3134. 1–17. https://doi.org/10.3390/ijerph18063134

Agyemang, C., Bhopal, R., & Bruijnzeels, M. (2005). Negro, Black, Black African, African Caribbean, African American or what? Labelling African origin populations in the health arena in the 21st century. *Journal of Epidemiology & Community Health, 59*(12), 1014–1018.

Ahonen, L., Loeber, R., & Brent, D. A. (2019). The association between serious mental health problems and violence: Some common assumptions and misconceptions. *Trauma, Violence, & Abuse, 20*(5), 613–625.

Alang, S., McAlpine, D., McCreedy, E., & Hardeman, R. (2017). Police brutality and black health: Setting the Agenda for public health scholars. *American Journal of Public Health, 107*(5), 662–665. https://doi.org/10.2105/AJPH.2017.303691

Aldrich, D. P., & Meyer, M. A. (2015). Social capital and community resilience. *American Behavioral Scientist, 59*(2), 1–16.

Allen, J. O., Watkins, D. C., Chatters, L., & Johnson-Lawrence, V. (2019). Mechanisms of racial health disparities: Evidence on coping and Cortisol from MIDUS II. *Journal of Racial and Ethnic Health Disparities, 7*, 207–216. https://doi.org/10.1007/s40615-019-00648-y

Amoah, P. A., Koduah, A. O., & Gyasi, R. M. (2018). "Who'll do all these if I'm not around?": Bonding social capital and health and well-being of inpatients. *International Journal of Qualitative Studies on Health and Well-being, 13*(1), 1–11.

Bennett, G. G., Merritt, M. M., Sollers Iii, J. J., Edwards, C. L., Whitfield, K. E., Brandon, D. T., & Tucker, R. D. (2004). Stress, coping, and health outcomes among African-Americans: A review of the John Henryism hypothesis. *Psychology & Health, 19*(3), 369–383.

Boeri, M., Gardner, M., Gerken, E., Ross, M., & Wheeler, J. (2016). "I don't know what fun is": Examining the intersection of social capital, social networks, and social recovery. *Drugs and Alcohol Today, 16*(1), 1–15.

Bourdieu, P. (1986). The forms of capital. In J. G. Richardson (Ed.), *The handbook of theory: Research for the sociology of education* (pp. 241–258). Greenwood Press.

Bowleg, L., Maria del Río-González, A., Mbaba, M., Boone, C. A., & Holt, S. L. (2020). Negative police encounters and police avoidance as pathways to depressive symptoms among US Black men, 2015–2016. *American Journal of Public Health, 110*(S1), S160–S166.

Brooks, M., Ward, C., Euring, M., Townsend, C., White, N., & Hughes, K. L. (2016). Is there a problem officer? Exploring the lived experience of black men and their relationship with law enforcement. *Journal of African American Studies, 20*(3), 346–362.

Brooms, D. R. (2020). Connecting with my Brothers: Exploring Black men's community, bonding and identities in college. *Gender and Education, 33*, 1–16.

Brooms, D. R., & Clark, J. S. (2020). Black misandry and the killing of Black Boys and Men. *Sociological Focus, 53*(2), 125–140.

Brooms, D. R., & Perry, A. R. (2016). "It's Simply Because We're Black Men" Black Men's experiences and responses to the killing of Black Men. *The Journal of Men's Studies, 24*(2), 166–184.

Cain, C. L., Wallace, S. P., & Ponce, N. A. (2017). Helpfulness, trust, and safety of neighborhoods: Social capital, household income, and self-reported health of older adults. *The Gerontologist, 58*(1), 1–11.

Campbell, F., & Valera, P. (2020). "The only thing new is the cameras": A Study of US College students' perceptions of Police violence on social media. *Journal of Black Studies, 51*(7), 654–670.

Coleman, J. S. (1988). Social capital in the creation of human capital. *American Journal of Sociology, 94*, S95–S121.

Coleman, J. S. (1990). *Foundations of Social Theory*. Harvard University Press.

Cone, J. (1986). *A Black theology of liberation*. Orbis Books.

Dean, L. T., Subramanian, S. V., Williams, D. R., Armstrong, K., Zubrinsky Charles, C., & Kawachi, I. (2015). Getting Black men to undergo prostate cancer screening: The role of social capital. *American Journal of Men's Health, 9*(5), 385–396.

Dickey, S. L., & Ogunsanya, M. E. (2018). Quality of life among Black prostate cancer survivors: An integrative review. *American Journal of Men's Health, 12*(5), 1648–1664.

Durr, M. (2015). What is the difference between slave patrols and modern day policing? Institutional violence in a community of color. *Critical Sociology, 41*(6), 873–879.

Franco-Paredes, C., Jankousky, K., Schultz, J., Bernfeld, J., Cullen, K., Quan, N. G., Krsak, M., Henao- Martínez, A. F., Krsak, M., & Kon, S. (2020). COVID-19 in jails and prisons: A neglected infection in a marginalized population. *PLoS Neglected Tropical Diseases, 14*(6), e0008409. https://doi.org/10.1371/journal.pntd.0008409

Franco-Paredes, C., Ghandnoosh, N., Latif, H., Krsak, M., Henao-Martinez, A. F., Robins, M., Vargas Barahona, L., & Poeschla, E. M. (2021). Decarceration and community re-entry in the COVID-19 era. *The Lancet Infectious Diseases, 21*(1), e10–e15. https://doi.org/10.1016/s1473-3099(20)30730-1

Galderisi, S., Heinz, A., Kastrup, M., Beezhold, J., & Sartorius, N. (2015). Toward a new definition of mental health. *World Psychiatry, 14*(2), 231–233.

Gilbert, K. L., Ray, R., Siddiqi, A., Shetty, S., Baker, E. A., Elder, K., & Griffith, D. M. (2016). Visible and invisible trends in black men's health: Pitfalls and promises for addressing racial, ethnic, and gender inequities in health. *Annual Review of Public Health, 37*, 295–311.

Goldstein, E., Benton, S. F., & Barrett, B. (2020). Health risk behaviors and resilience among low-income, black primary care patients: Qualitative findings from a Trauma-Informed Primary Care Intervention Study. *Family & Community Health, 43*(3), 187–199.

Gonzales, E., Gordon, S., Whetung, C., Connaught, G., Collazo, J., & Hinton, J. (2021). Acknowledging systemic discrimination in the context of a pandemic: Advancing an anti-racist and anti-ageist movement. *Journal of Gerontological Social Work*, 1–15.

Graham, P. W., Yaros, A., Lowe, A., & McDaniel, M. S. (2017). Nurturing environments for boys and men of color with trauma exposure. *Clinical Child and Family Psychology Review, 20*(2), 105–116.

Griffith, D. M. (2012). An intersectional approach to men's health. *Journal of Men's Health, 9*(2), 106–112.

Griffith, D. M. (2016). Biopsychosocial approaches to men's health disparities research and policy. *Behavioral Medicine, 42*(3), 211–215.

Griffith, D. M. (2018). "Centering the margins": Moving equity to the center of men's health research. *American Journal of Men's Health, 12*(5), 1317–1327.

Griffith, D. M., Metzl, J. M., & Gunter, K. (2011a). Considering intersections of race and gender in interventions that address US men's health disparities. *Public Health, 125*(7), 417–423.

Griffith, D. M., Ober Allen, J., & Gunter, K. (2011b). Social and cultural factors influence African American men's medical help seeking. *Research on Social Work Practice, 21*(3), 337–347.

Griffith, D. M., Bergner, E. M., Fair, A. S., & Wilkins, C. H. (2021a). Using mistrust, distrust, and low trust precisely in medical care and medical research advances health equity. *American Journal of Preventive Medicine, 60*(3), 442–445.

Griffith, D. M., Jaeger, E. C., Semlow, A. R., Ellison, J. M., Bergner, E. M., & Stewart, E. C. (2021b). Individually tailoring messages to promote African American Men's health. *Health Communication,* 1–10. https://doi.org/10.1080/10410236.2021.1913837

Harley, A. E., Frazer, D., Weber, T., Edwards, T. C., & Carnegie, N. (2020). No longer an island: A social network intervention engaging black men through CBPR. *American Journal of Men's Health, 14*(2), 1–13.

Harvey, I. S. (2013). The role of spirituality and Africana womanism in the self-management of chronic conditions among older African Americans. *Journal of Nursing Education and Practice, 3*(12), 81–92.

Hill, A. (2020). Free Speech v. Free Blacks: Racist policing and calls to harm. *First Amendment Studies, 54,* 1–7.

Hussen, S. A., Jones, M., Moore, S., Hood, J., Smith, J. C., Camacho-Gonzalez, A., del Rio, C., & Harper, G. W. (2018). Brothers building brothers by breaking barriers: Development of a resilience-building social capital intervention for young black gay and bisexual men living with HIV. *AIDS Care, 30*(sup4), 51–58.

Hutto, J. W., Sr., & Green, R. D. (2016). Social movements against racist Police brutality and Department of Justice Intervention in Prince George's County, Maryland. *Journal of Urban Health: Bulletin of the New York Academy of Medicine, 93*(Suppl 1), 89–121. https://doi.org/10.1007/s11524-015-0013-x

Jackson, A. N., Butler-Barnes, S. T., Stafford, J. D., Robinson, H., & Allen, P. C. (2020). "Can I Live": Black American Adolescent Boys' reports of Police abuse and the role of religiosity on mental health. *International Journal of Environmental Research and Public Health, 17*(12), 1–16.

Jacobs, L. A., Kim, M. E., Whitfield, D. L., Gartner, R. E., Panichelli, M., Kattari, S. K., Downey, M. M., McQueen, S. S., & Mountz, S. E. (2021). Defund the police: Moving towards an anti-carceral social work. *Journal of Progressive Human Services, 32*(1), 37–62.

James, S. A. (1994). John Henryism and the health of African-Americans. *Culture, Medicine, and Psychiatry, 18,* 163–182.

Jang, E., & Canada, K. E. (2014). New directions for the study of incarcerated older adults: Using social capital theory. *Journal of Gerontological Social Work, 57*(8), 858–871.

Johnson, O., Jr., Vil, C. S., Gilbert, K. L., Goodman, M., & Johnson, C. A. (2019). How neighborhoods matter in fatal interactions between police and men of color. *Social Science & Medicine, 220,* 226–235.

Johnson-Lawrence, V., Griffith, D. M., & Watkins, D. C. (2013). The effects of race, ethnicity, and mood/anxiety disorders on the chronic physical health conditions of men from a national sample. *American Journal of Men's Health, 7*(4_suppl), 58S–67S.

Kim, M. E. (2020). Anti-carceral feminism: The contradictions of progress and the possibilities of counter-hegemonic struggle. *Affilia, 35*(3), 309–326.

Lin, N. (1999). Building a network theory of social capital. *Connections, 22*(1), 28–51.

Lincoln, K. D., Taylor, R. J., Watkins, D. C., & Chatters, L. M. (2011). Correlates of psychological distress and major depressive disorder among African American men. *Research on Social Work Practice, 21*(3), 278–288.

Lopes, G. B., James, S. A., Lopes, M. B., Penalva, C. C., Silva, C. T. J. E., Matos, C. M., Martin, M. T. S., & Lopes, A. A. (2018). John Henryism and perceived health among hemodialysis patients in a Multiracial Brazilian Population: The PROHEMO. *Ethnicity & Disease, 28*(4), 539–548.

McGee, T. (2021). An era of new policing: Exploring the defunding of the Police. *FAU Undergraduate Law Journal*, 151–160.

Moore, S. E., Robinson, M. A., Adedoyin, A. C., Brooks, M., Harmon, D. K., & Boamah, D. (2016). Hands up—Don't shoot: Police shooting of young Black males: Implications for social work and human services. *Journal of Human Behavior in the Social Environment, 26*(3-4), 254–266.

Motley, R. O., Jr., Chen, Y. C., Johnson, C., & Joe, S. (2020). Exposure to community-based violence on social media among Black male emerging adults involved with the criminal justice system. *Social Work Research, 44*(2), 87–97.

Mrozla, T., Huynh, C., & Archbold, C. A. (2021). What took you so long? An examination of reporting time and Police misconduct complaint dispositions. *Deviant Behavior*, 1–15. https://doi.org/10.1080/01639625.2021.1919497

Nguyen, A. W., Chatters, L. M., & Taylor, R. J. (2016). African-American extended family and church-based social network typologies. *Family Relations, 65*(5), 701–715.

Nguyen, A. W., Taylor, R. J., Chatters, L. M., & Hope, M. O. (2019a). Church support networks of African Americans: The impact of gender and religious involvement. *Journal of Community Psychology, 47*(5), 1043–1063.

Nguyen, A. W., Taylor, R. J., Taylor, H. O., & Chatters, L. M. (2019b). Objective and subjective social isolation and psychiatric disorders among African Americans. *Clinical Social Work Journal, 48*, 1–12.

Nuzzo, J. L. (2020). Men's health in the United States: A national health paradox. *The Aging Male, 23*(1), 42–52.

Nyqvist, F., Pape, B., Pellfolk, T., Forsman, A. K., & Wahlbeck, K. (2014). Structural and cognitive aspects of social capital and all-cause mortality: A meta-analysis of cohort studies. *Social Indicators Research, 116*(2), 545–566.

Obasogie, O. K., & Newman, Z. (2017). Police violence, use of force policies, and public health. *American Journal of Law & Medicine, 43*(2-3), 279–295.

Ortiz, J. M., & Jackey, H. (2019). The system is not broken, it is intentional: The prisoner reentry industry as deliberate structural violence. *The Prison Journal, 99*(4), 484–503.

Parker, L. (2015). Critical race theory in education and qualitative inquiry: What each has to offer each other now? *Qualitative Inquiry, 1*(7), 1–6.

Pew Research Center. (2019). *Facts About the U.S. Black Population*. Retrieved from https://www.pewresearch.org/social-trends/fact-sheet/facts-about-the-us-black-population/

Pitas, N., & Ehmer, C. (2020). Social Capital in the Response to COVID-19. *American Journal of Health Promotion, 34*(8), 942–944.

Preston, S. A. (2021). Abolitionist disjuncture: Reducing police violence in frontline social work. *Intersectionalities: A Global Journal of Social Work Analysis, Research, Polity, and Practice, 9*(1), 142–153.

Prost, S. G., Novisky, M. A., Rorvig, L., Zaller, N., & Williams, B. (2021). Prisons and COVID-19: A desperate call for gerontological expertise in correctional health care. *The Gerontologist, 61*(1), 3–7.

Putnam, R. D. (1993). *Making democracy work*. Princeton University Press.

Putnam, R. D. (1995). Bowling alone: America's declining social capital. *Journal of Democracy, 6*, 65–78.

Richie, B. E., & Martensen, K. M. (2020). Resisting carcerality, embracing abolition: Implications for feminist social work practice. *Affilia, 35*(1), 12–16.

Richmond, T. S., Wiebe, D. J., Reilly, P. M., Rich, J., Shults, J., & Kassam-Adams, N. (2019). Contributors to Postinjury mental health in urban black men with serious injuries. *JAMA Surgery, 154*(9), 836–843.

Robinson, M. A., Jones-Eversley, S., Moore, S. E., Ravenell, J., & Adedoyin, A. C. (2018). Black male mental health and the Black church: Advancing a collaborative partnership and research agenda. *Journal of Religion and Health, 57*(3), 1095–1107.

Santee, E. J., King, K. A., Vidourek, R. A., & Merianos, A. L. (2018). Health-related quality of life social determinants impacting African-American cancer survivors: A secondary data analysis of the 2014 behavioral risk factor surveillance system. *American Journal of Health Studies, 33*(1), 11–20.

Sickel, A. E., Seacat, J. D., & Nabors, N. A. (2019). Mental health stigma: Impact on mental health treatment attitudes and physical health. *Journal of Health Psychology, 24*(5), 586–599.

Smith, E., & Hattery, A. J. (2010). African American Men and the Prison Industrial Complex. *Western Journal of Black Studies, 34*(4), 387–398.

Smith, J., Griffith, D., White, A., Baker, P., Watkins, D., Drummond, M., & Semlow, A. (2020). COVID-19, equity and men's health. *International Journal of Men's Social and Community Health, 3*(1), e48–e64.

Snowden, L. R., & Graaf, G. (2021). COVID-19, social determinants past, present, and future, and African Americans' health. *Journal of Racial and Ethnic Health Disparities, 8*(1), 12–20.

Solórzano, D., Ceja, M., & Yosso, T. (2000). Critical race theory, racial microaggressions, and campus racial climate: The experiences of African-American college students. *Journal of Negro Education, 69*, 60–73.

Staggers-Hakim, R. (2016). The nation's unprotected children and the ghost of Mike Brown, or the impact of national police killings on the health and social development of African American boys. *Journal of Human Behavior in the Social Environment, 26*(3-4), 390–399.

Stern, M. F., Piasecki, A. M., Strick, L. B., Rajeshwar, P., Tyagi, E., Dolovich, S., Patel, P. R., Fukunaga, R., & Furukawa, N. W. (2021). Willingness to receive a COVID-19 vaccination among incarcerated or detained persons in correctional and detention facilities—Four states, September–December 2020. *Morbidity and Mortality Weekly Report, 70*(13), 473–477.

Taylor, R. J., & Chatters, L. M. (2010). Importance of religion and spirituality in the lives of African Americans, Caribbean Blacks and non-Hispanic Whites. *The Journal of Negro Education, 79*, 280–294.

Taylor, R. J., Chatters, L. M., & Brown, R. K. (2014). African-American religious participation. *Review of Religious Research, 56*(4), 513–538.

Taylor, R. J., Chatters, L. M., Lincoln, K. D., & Woodward, A. T. (2017). Church-based exchanges of informal social support among African Americans. *Race and Social Problems, 9*(1), 53–62.

Thorpe, R. J., & Whitfield, K. E. (2018). Psychosocial influences of African Americans Men's Health. *Journals of Gerontology: Psychological Sciences, 73*(2), 185–187. https://doi.org/10.1093/geronb/gbx125

Turner-Musa, J., Ajayi, O., & Kemp, L. (2020). Examining social determinants of health, stigma, and COVID-19 disparities. *Healthcare (Basel), 8*(2), E168.

U.S. Census Bureau. (2016). *Defining rural at the U.S. census bureau: American community survey and geography brief (Report No. ACSGEO-1)*. Retrieved from https://www2.census.gov/geo/pdfs/reference/ua/Defining_Rural.pdf

Verduin, F., Smid, G. E., Wind, T. R., & Scholte, W. F. (2014). In search of links between social capital, mental health and sociotherapy: A longitudinal study in Rwanda. *Social Science & Medicine, 121*, 1–9.

Watkins, D. C., Walker, R. L., & Griffith, D. M. (2010). A meta-study of Black male mental health and well-being. *Journal of Black Psychology, 36*(3), 303–330.

Watkins, D. C., Hudson, D. L., Howard Caldwell, C., Siefert, K., & Jackson, J. S. (2011). Discrimination, mastery, and depressive symptoms among African American men. *Research on Social Work Practice, 21*(3), 269–277.

Watkins, D. C., Assari, S., & Johnson-Lawrence, V. (2015). Race and ethnic group differences in comorbid major depressive disorder, generalized anxiety disorder, and chronic medical conditions. *Journal of Racial and Ethnic Health Disparities, 2*(3), 385–394.

Westerhof, G. J., & Keyes, C. L. (2010). Mental illness and mental health: The two continua model across the lifespan. *Journal of Adult Development, 17*(2), 110–119.

Williams, J. M. (2017). Race and justice outcomes: Contextualizing racial discrimination and Ferguson. *Ralph Bunche Journal of Public Affairs, 6*(1), 1–7.

Williams, J. M. (2019). Race as a carceral terrain: Black lives matter meets reentry. *The Prison Journal, 99*(4), 387–395.

Williams, J. M., Wilson, S. K., & Bergeson, C. (2019). "It's hard out here if you're a Black felon": A critical examination of Black male reentry. *The Prison Journal, 99*(4), 437–458.

Williams, J. M., Wilson, S. K., & Bergeson, C. (2020). Health implications of incarceration and reentry on returning citizens: A qualitative examination of Black Men's experiences in a Northeastern City. *American Journal of Men's Health, 14*(4), 1–16.

Xanthos, C., Treadwell, H. M., & Holden, K. B. (2010). Social determinants of health among African–American men. *Journal of Men's Health, 7*(1), 11–19.

Zhang, J., & Lu, N. (2019). What matters most for community social capital among older adults living in urban China: The role of health and family social capital. *International Journal of Environmental Research and Public Health, 16*(4), 558.

Raymond Adams, PhD, MSW, is Associate Professor of Social Work with tenure within the College of Education, Humanities, and Behavioral Sciences at Alabama A&M University in Huntsville, Alabama in the Department of Social Work, Psychology, and Counseling. Raised in Monroe, Louisiana, he has earned a Bachelor of Psychology degree from the University of Louisiana at Monroe in Spring 2006, a Master of Social Work degree from Baylor University in the Spring of 2011, and a Doctor of Philosophy in Social Work from Jackson State University in Spring 2019. His research centers on addressing issues of prostate cancer (PrCA) survivorship specifically as it relates to investigating the nexus between mental health, social networks, and spirituality among older, rural African American PrCA survivors. At the 65th CSWE APM in Denver, Colorado, for his publication entitled "Louisiana Black Men at risk for prostate cancer: An Untold Autoethnography" in the *Journal of Social Work and Christianity,* he was awarded the CRECD (Council on Racial, Ethnic, and Cultural Diversity) Award for PhD Candidates. Moreover, he was awarded the inaugural Frederick Douglass Teaching Scholars Fellowship at West Chester University's Graduate Social Work program in July 2019, where he became the inaugural Frederick Douglass Teaching Fellow teaching a 3-credit hour graduate course for the Graduate Social Work Department. Presently, he is an online MPH graduate student in Jiann-Ping Hsu College of Public Health at Georgia Southern University and serves as a Board Member on the Editorial Board for the *Journal of Social Work and Public Health.* He provides consultation to community organizations, religious institutions, and educational institutions on the impact of their healthcare policies and culturally-informed interventions on older African and African American men and their families. He is most proud of his role as uncle to Kharion, AJ, and the newest addition, Cairo Ifechi Nmeka, and godfather to Abdoulaye N'diaye.

Chapter 2
Black Men and Healthy Together: Self-Management of Chronic Disease and Behavioral Health

Evelina Sterling, Vanessa Robinson-Dooley, Carol Collard, and Tyler Collette

Maintaining a healthy lifestyle is one method to increase life expectancy. However, particular groups in America are at a disadvantage in terms of being healthy, from accessing health care to eating the right food. As a result, these individuals are more likely to suffer from chronic diseases and live shorter lives. African Americans, for example, are twice as likely to suffer from blindness as a result of diabetes than Caucasians/White Americans (Collins-McNeil et al., 2012; Sherman et al., 2019). African Americans are also at an increased risk of heart failure (Hughes & Granger, 2014). Specifically, Black/African American men in the United States are disproportionately suffering from chronic illnesses such as diabetes, hypertension or high blood pressure (HBP), cancer, and arthritis (Esiaka et al., 2019). Thus, this community must secure the proper and focused recognition it deserves through education about barriers to health and proven techniques that provide the skills and

E. Sterling
Department of Sociology & Office of Research, Kennesaw State University, Kennesaw, GA, USA
e-mail: esterlin@kennesaw.edu

V. Robinson-Dooley (✉)
School of Social Work, Simmons University, Boston, MA, USA
e-mail: vanessa.robinson-dooley@simmons.edu

C. Collard
Department of Social Work and Human Services, Kennesaw State University, Kennesaw, GA, USA
e-mail: ccollard@kennesaw.edu

T. Collette
Office of Research, Kennesaw State University, Kennesaw, GA, USA
e-mail: tcollet1@kennesaw.edu

© The Author(s), under exclusive license to Springer Nature Switzerland AG 2022
Y. D. Dyson et al. (eds.), *Black Men's Health*,
https://doi.org/10.1007/978-3-031-04994-1_2

knowledge necessary for taking control of one's preventative health. The purpose of such efforts is to consider the life experiences of this population carefully and supporting literature to develop a peer-led self-management program with competencies specific to African American men.

Black Men and Chronic Disease

Recent research has highlighted the state of African Americans as it relates to chronic illnesses or diseases. This recent focus is, of course, beneficial for scholars because it provides a new lens through which we can evaluate the current circumstances affecting this community. For instance, Dubbin et al. (2017) informed readers that for the African Americans who participated in their study, coronary heart disease (CHD) is considered a "Black disease." A Black disease is a racially disparate disorder where the onset of the illness is perceived as a normative experience for those who develop it.

Furthermore, African Americans who suffer from CHD relate the illness directly to poor diet and high-risk behaviors due to ongoing racial and socio-structural dynamics in which their health burdens form, sustain, and reproduce. The results presented by Dubbin's research team provide scholars with the personal experiences and perceptions of African Americans in America regarding their health. Other chronic diseases that this community face include diabetes, psoriasis, osteoporosis, pain, arthritis, cancer, ulcers, and cardiovascular diseases that encompass CHD, stroke, heart failure, and HBP (Esiaka et al., 2019; Griffith, 2015; Hughes & Granger, 2014; Marshall, 2014; Veenstra, 2012). However, most of this literature is not specific to Black men. The resulting gap in our understanding of how to best address this community's population-specific issues requires correction. It is clear that more research dedicated to this community is necessary to understand unique issues, burdens, and perspectives related to African American men.

Research that has focused on African American men regarding health disparities is emphasized in recent literature. Allen et al. (2019) found that midlife and older Black men display signs of poor physical and mental health and early mortality compared to white men of the same age. Additionally, Black men were more susceptible to negative health outcomes associated with blunted diurnal cortisol slopes, linked to poor mental and physical health and early mortality. While the research was limited to a small sample size that could hinder its external validity, it provides specific data on the health of African American men in the United States often underrepresented in literature.

Earlier work by Bond and Herman (2016) echo Allen et al.'s (2019) call for more focused research on African American men's mortality and life expectancy. According to Bond and Herman (2016), Black men continue to have a substantially lower life expectancy than Black women and white men and women. They report a disturbing lag in the increases in the likelihood of survival between 45 and 75 years old for Blacks, the most significant gap in survival belonging to Black men. They are also far behind in terms of insurance coverage and access to adequate health care. This evidence further emphasizes the need to evaluate Black men as a unique group, with distinct issues even within their racial community. In terms of achieving the goal of a healthy lifestyle, Black men appear to be so far behind, in part, due to lower life expectancy. Additionally, there are historical, social, economic, physical, and biological risk factors that define the Black male experience in America and contribute to increased rates of early morbidity and mortality (e.g., spaces where Black men and their families live, work, worship, and play; family formulation in the Black community; and individual social, economic, and behavioral risk that come with simply being Black in America). The disadvantages only serve to decrease the likelihood of Black men being included in health programs. In fact, efforts to eliminate these inequities have failed to include methods or interventions to improve Black men's health (Bond & Herman, 2016; Cole et al., 2014). While Cole and colleagues, specifically, conducted a location-based study in New York City that cannot be generalizable to other parts of the country, the information provided by this literature is beneficial to and helpful for scholars who wish to understand a population that is rarely mentioned in studies.

Self-Management

When struggling with chronic disease diagnoses, learning ways to reduce "flare-ups" is beneficial and vital to healthy living. It is for this reason that utilizing self-management is necessary, especially for the African American community. Research has highlighted barriers to self-management, including medication side effects, unhealthy eating, and fears related to a specific diagnosis (Long et al., 2017; Sherman & Williams, 2018). Within the African American community, self-management programs tailored specifically for Black men are rare. Jack and colleagues (2010) noted that research for diabetes self-management, for example, typically focuses on Black women. As such, this gap in concentration indicates a desperately needed, carefully designed, self-management education and intervention program for African American men.

In very basic terms, self-management can be described as managing or tackling one's health diagnosis (i.e., reducing the likelihood of worsening symptoms) by themselves. It can also be described as a treatment that focuses on teaching individual problem-solving skills and increasing the skill set of the patient rather than simply offering information (Bodenheimer et al., 2002; Clark et al., 2008). Although the self-management discussed below is not modified to accommodate the needs of our target population, the research provides working definitions of self-management that highlight the unique benefits of self-management education over traditional patient education. This foundation is an asset for developing a self-management program for Black men.

Self-management creates self-efficacy (Bodenheimer et al., 2002). Self-efficacy plays an essential role in self-management. Researchers Katch and Mead (2010) reviewed effective cardiovascular disease self-management programs. For this review, each program recognized the impact that self-efficacy can have on a patient's adherence to treatment and their ability to manage their diagnosis. Another commonality among the programs was a multidisciplinary approach in the development. Utilizing this approach appeared to show an improvement in patients' self-efficacy by reaching them at their current status (equivalent to social work's notion of meeting the client where they're at) and applying the material to their individual needs. This review provided advantageous knowledge on the importance of self-management as it relates to health. With this information, we know that there appears to be a link between self-management, self-efficacy, and increased healthy behaviors.

Self-Management Programs

In the literature, there is research on self-management programs and their effectiveness with particular populations. Hawkins (2019), for example, reviewed the current state of literature for self-management programs for non-Hispanic Black men with type 2 diabetes (T2D). In these programs, the interventions led to increased knowledge of T2D self-management, exercise, visits to the primary care doctor, and improvements in clinical outcomes such as blood pressure and weight. Additionally, it was reported that Black men prefer intervention delivery to be outside of the traditional clinical setting and in places where they feel comfortable, topics of discussion relevant to them (e.g., T2D education, complications, exercise, and diet), and situating the content to be situationally and culturally appropriate while considering their work and life when scheduling. Hawkins's review provided scholars with vital personal preferences valued by the population of focus essential for developing a novel, targeted, program. However, as noted previously, like many others, research on Black men is scarce.

Katch and Mead (2010), as noted earlier, discussed five self-management programs. The most notable were the programs conducted by Lorig and colleagues. The first program consisted of the use of the self-efficacy theory to improve disease management. It was a seven-week program with weekly two and a half hour sessions on topics such as adopting exercise programs; using cognitive symptom management techniques; changing dietary habits; adhering to medication; using available community resources; managing fear, anger, and depression; and training(s) on effective communication with health professionals. After one year, the results showed a significant reduction in health distress, fewer visits to physicians and the emergency department, and increased perceived self-efficacy. Also, there was reduced utilization in services after one year, which was associated with higher levels of self-efficacy.

The second program developed by Lorig and colleagues, discussed in Katch and Mead (2010), was created for Spanish-speaking patients. The goal was to improve patient self-efficacy through a community-based program for Spanish-speaking individuals with chronic diseases, including heart disease. The program was a 14-hour community-based program presented in two and a half hour sessions over six weeks. It was made to be culturally and linguistically appropriate for the participants. The results of this program showed an improvement in participants' self-efficacy, healthy behaviors, and health status four months after the completion of the program.

A program called "Women Take PRIDE" was developed and based on an earlier chronic disease self-management intervention titled "Take PRIDE." This program was designed to enhance the overall disease self-management among women aged 60 years and older diagnosed with cardiovascular disease. Groups of 6–8 participants completed two and a half hours of instruction for four consecutive weeks. The self-management was different for each participant, as it was based on a heart regimen provided by their physician and was an area that was problematic for them. The results indicated a 46% decrease in hospital inpatient days, 49% decrease in inpatient charges, 41% decrease in heart-related hospital admission, and 61% decrease in inpatient days (Katch & Mead, 2010).

The fourth self-management program discussed in the Katch and Mead (2010) review examined the effect of cardiac rehabilitation (CR) on exercise self-efficacy, motivational readiness for exercise, and decisional balance for exercise adoption for patients with cardiovascular disease. A transtheoretical model of motivational readiness, which conceptualizes behavior change through a progression of "stages" of readiness, was utilized along with a twelve-week exercise regimen administered by a nurse, an exercise physiologist, and a cardiologist. Participants met three times a week for one hour and fifteen minutes and weekly for educational classes on medication management, cardiac risk factors, guidelines for home activity, stress management, and nutrition planning. The results indicated that CR produced significant gains in both exercise self-efficacy and motivational readiness for exercise, increased self-efficacy for exercise and the time spent exercising, and a reduction in overall ratings of barriers to exercise.

The final self-management program in the Katch and Mead (2010) review was a disease management program developed for low literacy patients with heart failure. The program consisted of a two-hour focus group of four patients and individual interviews with four other patients. The educational material used in this program was modified for appropriateness (i.e., a picture-based educational booklet with simple language). The results of this program indicated a self-reported 100% of participants weighed themselves every day or several times a week twelve weeks after the program. Additionally, there was a decrease in heart failure symptoms after three months.

Although they may not have been specific to Black men, for each program in which Katch and Mead reviewed, the programs provided accommodation of some sort in order to make it appropriate to their population of focus. Accommodations were a commonality among the five programs, to be a vital piece of an effective self-management program for chronic disease. However, it is essential to note the limitations within these results. Most programs were conducted voluntarily, influencing the results if patients already had a high level of self-efficacy.

Preliminary Support for this Culturally Competent Self-Management Program

The PI for the currently funded R15 AREA grant study, Dr. Sterling, served as a health education expert and evaluation consultant in developing the curriculum for the Health and Recovery Peer (HARP) Program, an adapted version of the Chronic Disease Self-Management Program (CDSMP), specifically targeting people with serious mental illness (SMI). The initial pilot testing of HARP (funded by NIMH R34MH078583) established its feasibility. It showed promise in improving a range of self-management and health outcome measures, including improvements in patient activation and greater likelihood of using primary care medical services. In terms of baseline characteristics, the mean age of the study population was 48; most were women (82.5%); a vast majority (82.5%) were African American, and most were poor (mean annual income $7704). A total of 20% of participants were uninsured, with the majority having Medicaid and/or Medicare. The most common primary mental diagnoses were bipolar disorder (32.5%), schizophrenia (28.8%), major depression (26.3%), and PTSD (11.3%). The most common medical comorbidities were hypertension (62.5%), arthritis (48.8%), asthma (22.5%), and heart disease (22.5%).

For the initial pilot study, a total of 80 subjects were randomized to either the HARP intervention (n = 41) or standard care (n = 39). Among those completing baseline assessments, 81.2% completed the 6-month follow-up. Participants in the intervention group attended a mean of 4.75 out of the six sessions. At 6-month follow-up, participants in the HARP program showed more remarkable improvement in patient activation than those in usual care (7.7% relative improvement vs. 5.7% decline, p = 0.03 for group*time interaction) and in rates of having one or more primary care (68.4% vs. 51.9% with one or more visit, p = 0.046 for group*time interaction). Intervention advantages were observed for physical health-related quality of life (HRQOL), physical activity, and medication adherence and, though not statistically significant, had similar effect sizes as those seen for the CDSMP in general medical populations. Improvements in HRQOL were the largest among medically and socially vulnerable subpopulations. This peer-led medical self-management program was feasible and showed promise for improving a range of health outcomes among mental health consumers with chronic medical comorbidities, particularly with more substantial curriculum adaptations.

Next, a multisite randomized trial of HARP was conducted with a total of 401 participants with an SMI and one or more chronic medical conditions across three community mental health clinics (funded by NIMH R01MH090584). Like the previous pilot study, most participants were female, African American, and/or poor; nearly all were uninsured or covered by public insurance. The most common psychiatric diagnoses were depression, bipolar disorder, and schizophrenia, and the most common chronic medical conditions were hypertension, hyperlipidemia, asthma, and diabetes. Assessments were conducted at baseline, three months, and six months. A total of 75.3% of participants in the intervention group attended at least 5 out of 6 sessions. At the 6-month follow-up, subjects in the intervention group (as compared with usual care) demonstrated improvements in the Physical Component Summary (2.7 vs. 1.4 point increase, p = 0.046) and Mental Component Summary (4.6 vs. 2.5 point increase, p = 0.039) of the SF-36. For secondary outcomes at 6-month follow-up, there were greater improvements for the intervention group for mental health recovery (p = 0.02), but no statistically significant differences for patient activation, dietary intake, medication adherence, or report of a usual source of medical care. As the first fully powered randomized trial of a peer-led intervention to address medical self-management in patients with SMI, the presented study provides compelling evidence that these programs hold the potential to improve the health and well-being of patients with serious mental illnesses. This study was the most extensive study of its kind. It is evident that with further adaptations and refinement of the self-management program, researchers can meet the needs of vulnerable and underserved populations specifically.

"Healthy Together"

With the information gathered from the literature available and our preliminary data, our goals are to: (1) outline a distinct need for a culturally competent self-management program for Black men with chronic illnesses, and (2) pilot a newly developed peer-led self-management program titled "Healthy Together." From the pilot study, in which the Stanford University's Chronic Disease Self-Management Program (CDSMP) and its effectiveness were reviewed, the results did not improve healthy behaviors or self-efficacy. There was an increase in overall activity, stretching, and equipment activity and a decrease in the number of days affected by poor mental and physical health; however, there were no significant results for increased self-efficacy. One potential reason for the nonsignificant results could be ascribable to cultural factors, further supporting the overall necessity for such programs and current research on the impact of appropriate program content for the population of focus (Collard et al., 2017). While the study is limited in external validity because of its small sample size, this pilot study did, however, add to the sparse research on Black men and provides some information and insight into how Black men can increase self-management through intercultural competence.

For this program, research will be conducted by gathering qualitative data from the target population, their families, and their healthcare providers to better describe their experience. A culturally appropriate peer-led self-management curriculum will be developed and reviewed by clinicians for medical accuracy using the previously described data. The curriculum will include a health coaching-type model led by peer facilitators (one-on-one focused self-management support program). It will combine the CDSMP and the Flinders Program to introduce case management and self-management support through health coaching to encourage systemic and organizational change to develop an integrated care plan for each participant. The use of technology will also be implemented via virtual meetings, electronic medication management, calendaring, symptom trackers, fitness and nutrition trackers, and journaling and personal health records as appropriate. Last, the curriculum will include mobile decision support, family involvement, and community resources to gain information and support to assist with managing chronic conditions.

The curriculum will be pilot tested in a nonexperimental design. At least 50 low-income Black/African American males who attended one of the four scheduled six-week peer-led interventions in both urban and rural settings will be enrolled in the program. The pilot will consist of a pre- and post-test to measure effectiveness. We will address attrition through over-enrollment and an intensive follow-up system. The follow-up will occur three months after the program assesses changes in knowledge, behaviors, health status, quality of life, self-efficacy, and patient activation. With the addition of culturally appropriate content for Black men, the hypothesis is that the results from this study will be more significant than the initial pilot study.

Summary

Previous research has outlined evident disparities in the development of chronic health conditions among African Americans compared to other groups, with African American men disproportionately affected by almost every disorder investigated. This chapter provides a succinct overview of the current state of the research on low-income African American men with chronic health conditions. It outlines the need for targeted, culturally competent programs designed to provide African American men the skills, resources, and tools useful for managing chronic conditions beyond the doctor's office. The authors argue that this community must be positioned with effective self-managed solutions to safeguard against worsening chronic conditions and maintaining effective strategies or preventative measures that result in positive health outcomes. The distinct goal of increasing the subjective and objective quality of life and improving life expectancies is of utmost importance to the authors.

Examinations into health conditions such as chronic heart disease (CHD) revealed that social determinants of health stemming from structural racism combined with cultural elements such as diet and risk-taking behaviors were highly related to the health burdens of African American men. Compounded by the fact that African American men are less likely to have access to adequate health insurance, a disturbing picture of health care emerges for many African American men. Yet, much literature exploring the experiences, expectations, and effects of chronic health conditions rarely focuses specifically on African American men.

Such a significant gap requires attention. Black men continue to have a substantially lower life expectancy than Black women and white men and women. The resulting disparity is a troublingly lower likelihood of survival between the ages of 45 and 75 years for African American men. Social determinants such as geographic location, employment, economic burdens, historical experiences, and biological predispositions decrease the likelihood of health programs including African American men in a targeted fashion. Moreover, attempts to reduce such injustices fail to embrace culturally competent techniques to improve Black men's health and quality of life. The authors propose that self-management programs can provide an agency-centered approach to health. Men can navigate their conditions more efficiently while promoting active and engaged strategies designed to improve their overall quality of life.

Self-management programs created explicitly for African American men are atypical and often do not involve the population of focus as collaborators in design. Broadly, self-management is the management of and attending to one's health diagnosis by the individual with the overt goal of reducing symptoms or preventing the condition from worsening. It is an intervention focused on teaching specific problem-solving skills, increasing proactive engagement, and providing techniques to achieve the stated goals above and beyond simple education. The resulting self-efficacy, defined agency, and valuable resources have improved health and subjective quality of life in other populations. However, the reported gap in concentration reveals a great need for a carefully designed self-management education and intervention program for African American men.

The authors provide favorable preliminary evidence in support of this need. Upon receiving a self-management intervention, African Americans in the treatment group exhibited improvements in patient activation, increased primary care, medication adherence, physical activity, and quality of life. These improvements were amplified in medically and socially vulnerable subpopulations. Similar improvements were observed in a follow-up study examining the effects of self-management on chronic mental health conditions. However, while these results are promising, African American men were substantially underrepresented.

"Healthy Together" is a novel program currently funded by the National Institutes of Health. It is designed to rectify the gap by combining researchers' understanding of the disparities experienced by economically and medically vulnerable African American men to the history and success of self-management programs deployed by the authors. It utilizes an often-neglected technique of integrating explicit experiences from the population of focus by conducted focus groups between the men themselves, their family members, and providers. The qualitative experiences will subsequently inform how the authors carefully adapt existing successful self-management interventions which reflect African American Men's experiences. With a culturally competent element employed in the intervention, the authors are optimistic that the improvements from preliminary studies will be magnified.

Discussion Questions
1. What has been your experience with males dealing with chronic disease? Discuss how that experience might be similar or different from the experience of the Black men discussed in this chapter. Discuss what factors might account for those differences and similarities.
2. Why would Black men be considered a vulnerable or underserved population when it comes to their health and health care? What do Black men have in common with other vulnerable or underserved populations? Explain how we can better support Black men's health.

3. What role, if any, do healthcare providers have in perpetuating disparities in health outcomes for minority populations? What can healthcare providers do to increase engagement and promote trust with Black male patients?

Exercises

1. Search the literature for information on chronic disease and Black males. Select one research article that discusses the impact of a chronic disease and Black men. Write a short reflection paper on ways that someone with this chronic disease can benefit from a self-management program like the one discussed in this chapter.
2. Look at the websites or other health education materials from major health organizations (e.g., American Heart Association, American Diabetes Association, American Cancer Society, etc.). How do these health organizations address the specific needs of Black men, especially since Black men are often disproportionately affected by chronic conditions and other health issues? Create new educational materials or messages that are more culturally appropriate and would better address the needs of Black men.
3. Search the literature for information on cultural differences in how patients interact with healthcare providers. Design a flyer promoting the opening of a health clinic in a low-income African American community. Based on your research, what would you include to encourage Black men to seek help?

Glossary of Terms and Concepts

Chronic Disease Self-Management: A health management program for individuals with at least one identified chronic health condition focused on providing patients with agency-centered skills, resources, and tools such as problem solving, decision-making, planning, and taking an active role in managing their chronic conditions.

Chronic Disease: Broadly defined, a chronic disease is a condition persisting for one year or longer which requires ongoing medical treatment or attention and causes limits to daily activities or a combination of both.

Mortality: The number of deaths among a particular demographic of people during a specified period of time.

Cultural Competence: Understanding the cultural elements of different peoples in need of social services with explicit focus on how to navigate differences in beliefs, value systems, traditions, or norms that are not familiar to the clinician.

Low Income: An individual or family in impoverished conditions due to the need to spend a greater proportion, roughly 20% more, of their income on essentials like shelter, clothing, and food than the average individual/family.

Health Disparity: Societal health characteristics resulting from the multifaceted interaction of numerous components such as environmental, individual differences, genetic, and social risk factors stemming from ubiquitous social determinants of health and structural inequities believed to be the principal cause.

Community Health: A public health field focused on examining, protecting, and improving health within a group of people who may differ on specific characteristics but share broad qualities such as values, goals, social interests, geographic location, ethnicity, or culture.

References

Allen, J. O., Watkins, D. C., Chatters, L., Geronimus, A. T., & Johnson-Lawrence, V. (2019). Cortisol and racial health disparities affecting black men in later life: Evidence from MIDUS II. *American Journal of Men's Health, 13*(4), 1557988319870969.

Bodenheimer, T., Lorig, K., Holman, H., & Grumbach, K. (2002). Patient self-management of chronic disease in primary care. *Innovations in Primary Care, 288*(19), 2469–2475.

Bond, M. J., & Herman, A. A. (2016). *Lagging life expectancy for black men: A public health imperative.*

Clark, D. O., Frankel, R. M., Morgan, D. L., Ricketts, G., Bair, M. J., Nyland, K. A., & Callahan, C. M. (2008). The meaning and significance of self-management among socioeconomically vulnerable older adults. *Journal of Gerontology, 63B*(5), S312–S319.

Cole, H., Schoenthaler, A., Braithwaite, S., Ladapo, J., Mentor, S., Uyei, J., & Trinh-Shevrin, C. (2014). *Community-based settings and sampling strategies: Implications for reducing racial health disparities among black men, New York City, 2010–2013.*

Collard, C., Robinson-Dooley, V., Patrick, F., & Farabaugh, K. (2017). Efficacy of chronic disease self-management among low-income black males with behavioral health disorders: Pilot study. *Georgia Public Health Association, 6*(4), 420–425.

Collins-McNeil, J., Edwards, C. L., Batch, B. C., Benbow, D., McDougald, C. S., & Sharpe, D. (2012). A culturally targeted self-management program for African Americans with type 2 diabetes mellitus. *The Canadian Journal of Nursing Research, 44*(4), 126–141.

Dubbin, L., McLemore, M., & Shim, J. K. (2017). Illness narratives of African Americans living with coronary heart disease: A critical interactionist analysis. *Qualitative Health Research, 27*(4), 497–508.

Esiaka, D., Naemi, P., Kuofie, A., & Hess, R. (2019). General well-being in adult black males with chronic illness. *Gerontology & Geriatric Medicine, 5*, 1–8.

Griffith, C. J. (2015). *Racial differences in the impact of a worksite wellness program on cardiovascular biomarkers* [Doctoral dissertation, Walden University].

Hawkins, J. M. (2019). Type 2 diabetes self-management in non-hispanic black men: A current state of the literature. *Current Diabetes Reports, 19*(3), 10.

Hughes, H. A., & Granger, B. B. (2014). Racial disparities and the use of technology for self-management in blacks with heart failure: A literature review. *Current Heart Failure Reports, 11*, 281–289.

Jack, L., Jr., Toston, T., Jack, N. H., & Sims, M. (2010). A gender-centered ecological framework targeting black men living with diabetes: Integrating a "masculinity" perspective in diabetes management and education research. *American Journal of Men's Health, 4*(1), 7–15.

Katch, H., & Mead, H. (2010). The role of self-efficacy in cardiovascular disease self-management: A review of effective programs. *Patient Intelligence, 2*(Default), 33–44.

Long, E., Ponder, M., & Bernard, S. (2017). Knowledge, attitudes, and beliefs related to hypertension and hyperlipidemia self-management among African-American men living in the southeastern United States. *Patient Education and Counseling, 100*(5), 1000–1006.

Marshall, V. J. (2014). *The influence of race/ethnicity and alcohol use on high blood pressure and diabetes* [Doctoral dissertation, Kent State University].

Sherman, L. D., & Williams, J. S. (2018). Perspectives of fear as a barrier to self-management in non-hispanic black men with type 2 diabetes. *Health Education & Behavior, 45*(6), 987–996.

Sherman, L. D., Comer-Hagans, D. L., & Pattin, A. J. (2019). Experiences with stress among African American men living with type 2 diabetes: A qualitative inquiry. *SAGE Open Nursing, 5*, 1–9.

Veenstra, G. (2012). Expressed racial identity and hypertension in a telephone survey sample from Toronto and Vancouver, Canada: Do socioeconomic status, perceived discrimination and psychosocial stress explain the relatively high risk of hypertension for Black Canadians? *International Journal for Equity in Health, 11*, 1–10.

Evelina Sterling, PhD, is a medical sociologist and public health researcher focused primarily on health equity. She has a PhD in sociology from Georgia State University and a master's degree in public health from the Johns Hopkins University. She is also a master certified health education specialist. Currently, she is Associate Professor of Sociology and the Director of Research Development Strategic Initiatives at Kennesaw State University in Kennesaw, Georgia.

Vanessa Robinson-Dooley, LCSW, CNP received her BA in Political Science from Spelman College in Atlanta, Georgia. She also holds a Master of Public Administration (MPA) from Drake University, and Master (MSW) and Doctor of Social Work from The University of Georgia. She is a Licensed Clinical Social Worker in the state of Georgia. Her direct practice (therapist) experience includes individual and family therapy, group work, and assessments. She has also worked in the area of domestic violence, program development, and community organizing. Dr. Robinson-Dooley's research focus includes factors surrounding chronic diseases and behavioral health in African American men, and promoting cultural competency in education and practice. She is Co-PI on a $700,000 NIH grant with two colleagues from Kennesaw State University in Kennesaw, Georgia, studying self-management of chronic disease and behavioral health for Black men and developing a peer-led curriculum. Dr. Robinson-Dooley is teaching courses on "teaching" and is an advocate of UDL (Universal Design for Learning) principles and technology use in the class-room. She has published in multiple journals and presented nationally on various topics related to her teaching and research.

Carol Collard, PhD, LMSW, is an associate professor in the Department of Social Work and Human Services at Kennesaw State University in Kennesaw, Georgia. Her teaching focuses on macro social work as well as foundation courses centered on ethics, social justice and diversity. Dr. Collard's varied research interests include studying the intersection of homelessness and behavioral health disorders, self-efficacy, chronic disease self-management and social entrepreneurship. Professionally, Dr. Collard has been involved in the nonprofit sector serving chronically homeless individuals and families. Currently, Dr. Collard is a co-investigator on a NIH-funded study on chronic disease self-management for low-income African American men.

Tyler Collette, PhD, received his PhD from the University of Texas at San Antonio, where he studied military and cultural health. During his time there, he served as methodologist and statisti-cian for the Latino Health Research Initiative, using his skills to explore health disparities in the area and developing community-based interventions. He has more than 10 years of experience working with diverse communities and exploring psychological phenomena cross-culturally. He is currently a Postdoctoral Fellow in the Office of Research at Kennesaw State University in Kennesaw, Georgia, working on various projects including assisting in developing a self-management curriculum for African American men with multiple chronic health conditions.

Chapter 3
Positionality and Unpacking Current Perspectives on Black Male Health Toward Transformative Action

Brian Culp

Analyzing the current health status of Black men in the United States reveals the need for transformative action. By most measures in comparison to men and women of every racial group, the health profile of Black men is characterized by a significantly higher rate of disease and premature death. Black males have higher mortality rates from medical conditions and higher preventable morbidity (Jones-Eversley et al., 2020). Watkins et al. (2017) note that Black men are 31% more likely to die from all types of cancer with lower five-year survival rates at each stage of cancer diagnosis. Further, Black men are more likely to be diagnosed with Type 2 diabetes, are 14 times more likely to experience kidney failure due to hypertension, have a 30% higher mortality rate due to cardiovascular disease, and have a 60% higher mortality rate from stroke compared to non-Hispanic white men (Watkins et al., 2017, p. 6).

Despite this data on the overall health outcomes of Black men, there is still a dearth of literature and perspectives that specifically focuses on mental health challenges of this population. This is unsurprising as research studies have traditionally viewed physical health as separate from mental health. Mental health as defined by the World Health Organization (2001) is a state of well-being where one realizes that his or her own abilities can cope with normal life stressors and he or she can engage in work productively and fruitfully and can contribute to his or her community (Ward & Mengesha, 2013). Mental disorders are "health conditions that are characterized by alterations in thinking, mood, and/or behavior that are associated with distress and/or impaired functioning" (CDC, 2021).

B. Culp (✉)
Department of Health Promotion and Physical Education, Kennesaw State University, Kennesaw, GA, USA
e-mail: bculp1@kennesaw.edu

Y. D. Dyson et al. (eds.), *Black Men's Health*,
https://doi.org/10.1007/978-3-031-04994-1_3

Roughly one in five Americans struggle with mental illness. African Americans are 20% more likely to have serious psychological distress than other groups. Depression is a common mental health problem in the United States, affecting more than 17 million people per year. Black depressive occurrences have been found to be more disabling, persistent, and resistant to treatment than those experienced by white persons (Hankerson et al., 2015). Suicide is the third leading cause of death among African Americans ages 15–24 years. Black men are four times more likely to die by suicide than Black women. Studies also show that African Americans are five times more likely than whites to be diagnosed with schizophrenia. Overall, the overdiagnosis of schizophrenia and the underutilization of appropriate treatment are complicated by misdiagnosis, trauma, and racism (Schwartz & Blankenship, 2014).

Watkins (2012) suggested that the complexities of mental disorders and how it intersects with race, culture, and gender norms is representative of an intricate phenomenon for Black males. Simply put, there is much more to uncover. For example, the risk factors associated with depression and its resultant consequences are poorly understood (Watkins et al., 2006). Ward and Mengesha (2013) in their literature review found only 19 empirical studies over a 25-year period that had a focus on African American men and depression. This is a significant disappointment when considering that the prevalence rate of depression in Black men is suggested to be between 5% and 10%. When assessing anxiety disorders, literature suggests that Black men are particularly vulnerable to depression and anxiety due to numerous pressures associated with achieving higher status in a society that refuses to acknowledge their existence (Williams, 2018).

As Thorpe and colleagues (2020) have noted, Black men in the United States have a poor mental health profile that is influenced by a mix of structural forces that work against their optimal health and well-being. They navigate unique environmental stressors that other groups do not face, such as racism which exposes them to trauma and other post-traumatic stressors, as they move from adolescence to adulthood (Williams, 2018). This includes high rates of poverty, unemployment, and underemployment and incarceration at much higher rates than men of other racial/ethnic groups (Jäggi et al., 2016). Further, Black men are the most common subpopulation in the United States to experience violence of any type in American communities. Thus, to improve mental health outcomes for Black men in a transformative fashion, it is necessary to acknowledge the existence of barriers and systems that persist into the present day. After addressing these areas, several frameworks will be reconsidered to help advance positive health outcomes for this population. For the purposes of this chapter, it is understood that the terms "Black" and "African American" are used interchangeably to reflect a social, political, and culturally constructed ethnic group identity affiliated with the African diaspora. The word "Black" will also be capitalized for this reason.

The Permanence of Discrimination and Racism

While a complete discussion of the history of racism in mental health is beyond the scope of this chapter, it is necessary to provide a brief account to help frame the information to follow. Well into the twenty-first century, there is irrefutable evidence that discriminatory practices undermine the success and health of Black men (Hargrove & Brown, 2015). Racism is deeply ingrained in the formal policies, practices, and institutions of American society and is integral to the understanding the Black experience in the United States. Along with the trauma of chattel slavery introduced by white European colonizers in 1619, Black people were also victimized by the pseudoscientific tenets of scientific racism. These beliefs positioned whites as the "master race" and allowed for the invalidation of Black emotionality and intelligence in lieu of an emphasis on physical talent. For example, in justifying the enterprise of slavery, Black men were noted as having a basic psychological orientation that left them uniquely equipped for bondage (Taylor et al., 2019). Chattel slavery also placed Black men in the position of being unable to fully participate in the role of a husband and father. Likewise, Utsey (1997) suggested that the brutality of race-based chattel slavery prohibited a Black man from the ability to serve as a provider for his family and a protector from the evils of slavery.

The 13th Amendment ratified in 1865 after the Civil War formally abolished chattel slavery, but political and social change did not radically impact the fortunes of Black people in America. From the late nineteenth century through 1968, slavery was replaced by the Black Codes and later Jim Crow laws that institutionalized economic, educational, and social disadvantages for Blacks. Over the years to follow, social ills in America became attributed to Black men during the Civil Rights movement.

Schizophrenia, once a condition attributed to white middle-class housewives in the 1930s, was reframed as a violent social disease that afflicted "Negro men" in the early 1960s. The struggle for Black liberation was also called into question and framed as a catalyst for Black male mental illness. In 1968, Protest Psychosis was identified as a condition by Bromberg and Simon which hypothesized that "liberation caused delusions, hallucinations, and violent projections in black men" (Metzl, 2009, p. 100). Protest Psychosis would later be identified as schizophrenia, a notable fact when considering the dire statistic that African American men are diagnosed with schizophrenia at a rate five times more than any other race (Gara et al., 2019).

Distrust of Health Care and Government Response to Crisis

The COVID-19 pandemic has been a painful reminder that Black communities across the United States have been subjected to a long history of contracting and dying from disease due to health inequities and racial injustice. The Tuskegee

Syphilis Experiment conducted by the US Public Health Service studied the progression of untreated syphilis in African American men from 1932 to 1972. As one of the best-known examples of medical racism, inhumanity, and deception, African American participants were told that they were receiving free health care from the federal government. In truth, they were infected with syphilis and subjected to false diagnostic protocols, ineffective treatments, and disguised placebos over a 40-year period. During the years of the study and well after the 1940s validation of penicillin as an effective cure for the disease, 128 participants would perish from syphilis or related complications (Wells & Gowda, 2020).

Genocide has been a reoccurring theme that has framed the narrative that Blacks should be weary of health care. Noting the rise in infections and deaths among African Americans during the AIDS crisis, members of the Black community in the early 1990s began to openly question whether the government was manufacturing HIV in the attempt to eliminate African Americans. In retrospect, public health officials during the 1980s were slow to admit that a problem existed and were even slower to react. Research well into the twenty-first century indicates that significant numbers of Black men still harbor negative views and expectations of their health providers. Further, these studies suggest that this mistrust is linked to dissatisfaction, noncompliance, and underuse of healthcare services (Clark, 1998).

State and local governments have routinely responded to national disasters in ineffective ways that have disproportionally affected Black populations. The effects of the 2005 Gulf coast hurricanes (particularly Katrina) on New Orleans and other coastal areas of Louisiana, Mississippi, and Alabama were catastrophic for Black people (Toldson et al., 2011). While whites and Blacks suffered during this crisis, Black people in the years after Katrina were more likely to be displaced and financially unable to recover due to the impact of social inequities. Anxiety disorders such as PTSD in addition to health problems stemming from untreated fears of anticipating "what might be next" have been observed in long-term studies of Black groups who have survived a natural disaster.

The Flint water crisis that occurred from 2014 to 2019 in Flint, Michigan, is an example of environmental racism that impacted a predominately Black and impoverished community. In April 2014, during a series of cost-cutting measures, the city decided to move to a new water servicer in Detroit. Until the new servicer went online, water from the Flint River was pumped to the city and treated first for coli bacteria with extra chlorine. The extra chlorine, without additional treatment, caused corrosion in the pipes that allowed lead to leak into the water supply. A host of physiological problems among the community were seen immediately that included lead poisoning, hair loss, and skin rashes. As with Katrina, people expressed concerns about the future while navigating mental health anxieties related to routines such as bathing and cooking.

Each of the prior examples of malpractice has unmistakably created what Terrell and Terrell (1981) described as a "cultural phenomenon" that exists for African Americans. This phenomenon inspires a reluctance in Black groups to truly believe the motives of whites at face value due to historical and contemporary experiences with racism and oppression. As Black men have contemplated help with mental health, they routinely acquire learned distrusts due to significant experiences and expectations of racism and discrimination, concerns about privacy, prior substandard care in the past, concerns about being used for experiments without their knowledge (i.e., Tuskegee, Henrietta Lacks), and an overall general mistrust of health service providers that still primarily reflect white norms and values.

Access to Mental Health Providers and Interpersonal Barriers

Research comparing mental health care across groups finds evidence of disparities that significantly impact Black populations. Intertwined in these disparities are barriers that specifically influence how Black men perceive, realize, and choose to address their personal mental health challenges. Across all populations, it has been postulated that before an individual seeks mental health services, they embark in a process of negotiation where they assess whether treatment is necessary, access feasibility and options for treatment, and ultimately decide to seek treatment (Motley & Banks, 2018). African American men are 50% less likely to receive mental health treatment than white men and do not seek mental health services from African American women. Studies have indicated that Black boys and men when given a psychiatric diagnosis will often fail to engage in services that could assist in rehabilitation, irrespective of if these are in outpatient, school-based, residential, or general community medical settings.

Further, there is stigma that is associated with mental health services for Black men that provides unrealistic expectations of what it means to be a man (Howard et al., 2012). Traditional definitions of masculinity frame men as individuals who are tough, competitive, athletic, decisive, violent, powerful, and aggressive (Thomas et al., 2015). For Black men, conforming to these norms for behavior can be particularly dangerous when considering the impact of racism, societal definitions of success, and negative attitudes toward blackness. Mahalik et al. (2006) suggest that Black men respond to these pressures and historical weights by choosing to be hyper-masculine, as they become immersed in their Black identity and reject negative portrayals of Blacks found in society. As a result, the mere implication of mental weakness is a threat to their own identity; so many Black males choose to be self-reliant, strong, and tough, so they are not labeled as "crazy" or "soft."

The Need for Cultural Humility and the Decentralization of Whiteness and in Mental Health Services

Since the nineteenth century, the biomedical model of medicine has dominated Western society and has emphasized biological factors over psychological, environmental, and social influences. In recent years, there has been increased advocacy for approaches to health that consider the unique elements of every person's identity. In the early 1980s, the concept of cultural competence was introduced to healthcare services and professional preparation programs. Cultural competence gained further support from leading institutions such as the Institute of Medicine and health philanthropies such as the Robert Wood Johnson Foundation (Greene-Moton & Minkler, 2020). In short, cultural competency broadly focuses on the ability of the health professional to improve health status of the patient by integrating culture into the clinical context. This is done by integration and transformation knowledge about individuals and groups of people into specific standards, policies, practices, and attitudes used in appropriate cultural settings to increase the quality of services, thereby producing better outcomes.

While a noble endeavor and still positively situated in the core of many programs that train health professionals, cultural competency has undergone dramatic critique. Scholars have suggested that one can never truly be competent and that use of the term "competence" gives too much power to one entity having all the answers (Murray-Garcia & Tervalon, 2014). Finally, cultural competency is described as a binary construct that implies that an individual either has this ability to interact with members of certain groups or they do not (Chavez, 2018; Greene-Moton & Minkler, 2020). Cultural humility a concept first penned by Tervalon and Murray-Garcia (1998) has regained traction in mental health as it is more intentional. It is a lifelong process of self-reflection and self-critique whereby the individual not only learns about another's culture but begins with a comprehensive examination of their own beliefs, assumptions, values, biases, and cultural identities (Kumagai & Lypson, 2009; Yeager & Bauer-Wu, 2013).

Tervalon and Murray-Garcia (1998) go on to state that cultural humility is "best defined not as a discrete end point but as a commitment and active engagement in a lifelong process that individuals enter into on an ongoing basis with patients, communities, colleagues, and with themselves" (p. 118). This process recognizes the dynamic nature of culture since cultural influences change over time and vary depending on location (Yeager & Bauer-Wu, 2013, p. 2). As people navigate through several cultures during a day and even differences in these cultures, it is more realistic to think of the individual as an ever-changing entity. For Black men, this shift from mere cultural competence to cultural humility could serve in significantly eliminating barriers to care and approaches that are centered in white perspectives (Kumagai & Lypson, 2009).

In commenting on whiteness and the need for Black mental health supports during COVID-19, King et al. (2021) decried current practices in medical training for demonstrating no accountability to the lived experiences of Black people. They liken current medical practice to "a colonial biomedical knee analogous to that which killed George Floyd, because it fails to see how it denies the life of Black people" (p. 93). Citing King and Gillard (2019), King et al. (2021) suggest that mental health professions remain in tribal zones and cultural camps that perpetuate cultural myths rooted in whiteness and colonialism. Meyer and Zane (2013) underscore this, explaining that the bulk of psychological training that therapists receive is based on white norms and beliefs, which can influence competency of non-Black therapists. Further, there has been much debate over the years regarding versions of the Diagnostic and Statistical Manual of Mental Disorders (DSM). The index does not account for cultural factors that influence symptomatology or diagnoses that speak to cultural issues such as racial discrimination or acculturation. This is in keeping with a history of training programs in counseling, psychology, and social work that rarely include the voices of health researchers, theorists, and practitioners (Poussaint, 2002; Samson, 2018).

Ultimately, King et al. (2021) cite the need for true equality in meeting the needs of Black communities through adoption of a joint conception of race and mental health through coproduction. This strategy provides room for the creation of an Afrocentric contribution to the current diagnostic framework in mental health. Not only will Black communities be improved through an intentional emphasis on decolonizing existing practices, but other transcultural, antiracist, and inclusive models could inevitably emerge. Co-productive methodologies could also inform the conceptualization of mental health for other marginalized populations. Finally, King and associates (2021) espouse that mental health services account for the experiences of Black people, by committing to the recruitment and retaining of Black mental health professionals. As alluded to previously, Black men often prefer talking to someone who looks like them that may better understand their experience as they address mental health challenges (Whaley, 2001).

From Invisibility to Transformation: Revisiting Three Frameworks to Support the Positive Mental Health of Black Men

Gilbert et al. (2016) used Ralph Ellison's award-winning *Invisible Man* to frame the lack of attention given to Black men in the arena of public health. This novel is used here to as it pertains to framing mental health for this group. In *Invisible Man,* the narrator's quest for freedom and self- identity in a society is defined by skin color. Invisibility is a main theme in the novel and occurs as the white people in the United States refuse to see the narrator as an individual but a stereotypical Black boy to be humiliated and made fun of (Tiwari, 2013). The narrator describes himself at the outset as "invisible" because people refuse to see him as anything more than an emotionless savage. Throughout the rest of his travels, the narrator witnesses the torture of Black boys made to fight each other for fake coins on an electrified rug, he sees poor Black women being sexually exploited by one of the trustees in his college, and he observes several other incidents that equate beauty and obedience to whiteness.

One of the more memorable moments in the novel is when the narrator is injured in a factory, loses consciousness, and finds himself imprisoned in a hospital. As the narrator drifts in and out of consciousness, he listens to the white doctors' conversation about whether to treat him through electric shock (to alleviate mental disorders), castration, or a lobotomy. During this, the narrator is asked by the doctors' questions relating to his identity to which he cannot respond to as he is suffering spasms. As the scene progresses and the narrator is subjected to more current from shock therapy, he hears the doctors casually remark "that he has rhythm" (a clear stereotypical reference to Black people) as his body is shaking because of being electrified. The narrator leaves the hospital demonstratively changed because of trauma. While he has a different outlook, the narrator does not fully trust it, feeling as he is in the "grip of an alien personality," in a world that is still unquestionably racist (Tiwari, 2013).

Ellison's imagery throughout the novel is powerful, but this episode encapsulates what we know about Black men and how they feel about mental health in a society that does not value their lives. When these men need help, health systems instead of addressing their needs would rather treat the symptom than engage in endeavors that will combat the root of the problem: institutional and system racism. If this is accurate as is suggested here, the question of "How can Black males move from invisibility to transformation?" is warranted. This question will be addressed briefly with a reexamination of Critical Race Theory, Spatial Justice, and the Capabilities Approach.

Critical Race Theory

Critical Race Theory (CRT) was first formulated in the field of legal studies after the civil rights movement of the 1960s to address continued structural inequalities in the United States. As related to psychological science and mental health practice, Volpe et al. (2019) suggest that CRT should be adopted as a theoretical framework in which racism and power are studied as impactful reasons for psychological phenomena. In the view of the authors, implementation of CRT has been rebuffed in lieu of dominant perspectives in the field of psychology that still advocate for neutral and objective approaches. Despite the numerous issues that afflict Black communities and the men in these communities, psychology has been slow to acknowledge that structural factors play out in racialized contexts (Brown, 2003; Volpe et al., 2019).

To this end, scholars who feel that CRT is a necessary framework for dismantling racial health disparities have advocated for an intersectional approach to CRT (Gillborn, 2015). Intersectionality, a concept that originated in law and Black feminist theory by Kimberlé Crenshaw (1989), is generally defined as an examination of "how interconnected social categorizations (i.e., race, class, gender, sexuality) contribute to specific systemic oppressions and discriminations experienced by an individual or group" (Culp, 2020, p. 8). This also involves an examination of economic and historical context and their intersections with identity. Future psychological research on mental health should incorporate an intersectional approach with a CRT framework to change current narratives on Black male mental health. This narrative is part of a larger narrative of the Black community that positions them as powerless, uneducated, and healthy (Volpe et al., 2019).

Spatial Justice

The expansion of communities has shifted more attention to the impact of placemaking. Placemaking is a multifaceted approach to the design and management of public spaces. In this process, focus is placed on a community's assets and potential for growth through wellness initiatives. Placemaking is no longer a trend but an established policy of many municipalities that is funded through public and private organizations. However, placemaking is political. Culp (2017) notes that "without understanding the importance of these spaces to the communities who use them, we risk destroying the significance and benefits of individual cultures, as well as historic, community, and personal spaces" (p. 148). Sociopolitical elements, such as conflict over access, equality, and inclusion, can also define what a place means to people (DiMasso et al., 2011). Indeed, for racialized minorities, these factors can have an impact on how they perceive the value of their bodies in these spaces.

Koh (2017) provided a scenario that is worth contemplating as it relates to Black men, asking "What would placemaking look like when Black lives matter?" Koh's commentary referenced a Washington, D.C., director of planning's thoughts on PARK(ing) Day, a worldwide event where citizens, artists, and activists collaborate to temporarily transform parking spaces usually reserved for cars into temporary public parks or displays of art or community. While the director believed that the event was a nice day for staff, he also wondered if five Black males would last 10 min if they took over a parking spot, had a barbecue, and listened to music on a normal day.

Koh's (2017) astute inquiry of who gets to "disrupt" the public space paradigm is certainly appropriate and timely. The lack of placemaking policies and other spatial injustices such as gentrification, cityhood movements, and the unjustified killings by police should be analyzed in relation to how these occurrences impact the mental health of Black boys and men. Research and rehabilitation programs must be willing to go to the places where Black men are to gain their knowledge and opinions on what strategies can best assist their communities. As identity is heavily tied to community in Black populations, mental health initiatives must understand the history and politics embedded in these areas.

Capabilities Approach

As previously mentioned, the tendency for mental health approaches is to consider Black groups from a deficit perspective. The Capabilities Approach is a flexible theoretical framework that is a normative approach to human welfare that centers on the true capability of persons to achieve their well-being rather than the idea that they have the right or freedom to do so (Sen, 2011). The focus is not only on how people function but on them having capability as a practical choice. Reasoning in this manner means that an individual could be deprived of their capabilities via ignorance, government oppression, the lack of finances, or false consciousness (Sen, 1999). Nussbaum (2000) outlined ten central capabilities that should be supported and obtainable for all individuals that include life, bodily health, senses imagination and thought, emotion, practical reason, affiliation, other species, play, and control over one's environment.

Selected literature on Black male identity formation and embodied trauma is necessary to contemplate here to clarify why this approach could have merit. Black males have long been conscious of their own dualities and double consciousness in a nation that has not met their basic needs, while it continues to abuse and oppress them from the "cradle to the grave" (Du Bois, 1999; Fanon, 1967). Butler (2010) espouses that socially constructed identities of Black males are merely performances that are rooted in negative and oppressive stereotypes forged from historical ideas regarding the Black body. Further, the process by which Black men have formulated their identities is heavily rooted in trauma. Sotero (2006) and Walters et al. (2011) suggest that groups subjected to the evils of colonialism, slavery, and genocide have a higher prevalence of disease for generations after the original trauma was inflicted. Because this trauma is too painful or difficult to confront, it becomes a psychological shield, whereby Black men use various means to disconnect from the reality of their situation. Therefore, it is critical to believe the stories of Black males, identify examples of Black excellence frequently, and promote an ethos that Black people have a purpose (i.e., Somebodiness-Thurman/King). When used with CRT and investigations on how space is produced in communities, the Capabilities Approach could shed light on the behaviors and desires of Black men while providing transformative mental health solutions.

Conclusion: The Way Forward

Despite growing interest in improving health disparities afflicting racialized minorities, the health of Black men consistently ranks lowest across all groups in the United States (Gilbert et al., 2016). Clearly, there is much work to do. As implied here, it will take a collective, intentional effort from researchers, practitioners, policy makers, and health organizations to improve the mental health of Black men in America. It is also the hope that this chapter challenges mental healthcare providers to take a more expansive approach to mental health issues that Black men face, as they encompass numerous, historical, institutional, and structural contexts.

Summary
Black men have one of the highest preventable mortality and morbidity rates in the United States. To improve upon this, it is essential that an intentional and sustained

focus on Black male mental health in communities include an understanding of historical perspectives, current psychosocial challenges, and multiple frameworks.

Discussion Questions
1. What do you see as the major barriers for Black men in getting adequate mental health care?
2. How do the following affect mental health care among Black men?

   - Trauma
   - Structural racism
   - Poverty
   - Lack of information
   - Community stigma about mental health
   - Media
   - Fear of health providers

3. How do we support young Black boys who may be too young to be able to adequately express verbally the worries and fears they may have about their lives in our current society?

Exercises
1. What are your thoughts about Du Bois' concept of "Double Consciousness"? Years after the initial introduction of the term, the relevance of the term still exists for many Black people trying to find their identity while reconciling a sense of two-ness. What does this term look like to you when considering the position of Black men and boys in American society? Do you feel that the feeling of double consciousness/two-ness can ever be reconciled or solved? If so, *how* and when, and if not, *why*?
2. Examine historical and current stereotypes associated with Black men and boys and compare them to how white men and boys are perceived in the United States. How would you strategize the creation of safe spaces for Black men and boys to express their fears, vulnerabilities, and desires without the fear of being ostracized? If you were asked, how would you help them seek mental health services in a way that empowers their decision-making?
3. This chapter mentions the lack of support that Black men may have in attempting to address their mental health challenges. In the conclusion, it is noted that a collective, intentional effort from researchers, practitioners, policy makers, and health organizations could be beneficial in serving the needs of this population. Take a brief inventory of the community that you spend the most time in. In your opinion, who are three to five key partners that can be enlisted in this endeavor? Provide a brief rationale for the entities you selected.
4. With a partner, provide a list of five pros and five cons of disclosing mental illness.
5. Reflect upon an example from popular culture of a situation where a Black man or boy struggled with challenges related to mental health. Provide your opinion of how the individual dealt with the challenges brought about by the episode. Do

you feel as if you would have addressed the situation differently? Why or why not?

Glossary of Terms and Concepts

Whiteness: Whiteness is essential to understand in dismantling institutional and structural barriers that keep Black males from seeking help for mental illness. At first glance, the use of the term *whiteness* can appear bold and accusatory (Lynch, 2018). Yet, whiteness is not synonymous with white people (Leonardo, 2009; Painter, 2010). As Du Bois (1920) notes, whiteness is erroneously considered a default position of power and an identity created and supported by historical practices, laws, socially developed constructs on race, standards of behavior, and falsehoods. Whiteness is not just a matter of biology but includes interpretations of class, labor, gender, beauty, sexuality, and how these intersect (Painter, 2010). Leonardo (2002) espouses that white people have the choice to participate in whiteness given that it is a social construct, and they should disown and disidentify with whiteness to fight for racial justice and equality.

Cultural Humility: A process of reflection and lifelong inquiry involving self-awareness of personal and cultural biases as well as awareness and sensitivity to significant cultural issues of others. Core to the process of cultural humility is the professional's deliberate reflection of her/his values and biases (Yeager & Bauer-Wu, 2013).

Double Consciousness: Double consciousness is a concept in social philosophy referring, originally, to a source of inward "two-ness" putatively experienced by African Americans because of their racialized oppression and devaluation in a white-dominated society. The idea is central to understanding the experiences of Black people living in post-slavery America. Additionally, double consciousness serves as an important framework for understanding the experiences of marginalized and oppressed groups.

Critical Race Theory: Critical Race Theory (CRT) is a framework that refers to a broad social scientific approach to the study of race, racism, and society. Essential to understanding the concept is the understanding that racism serves as a systemic feature of social structure, not just individual actions that promote prejudice and bigotry. In CRT, race is at the center of analysis. Those who use this framework interrogate policies and practices that are taken for granted to uncover the overt and covert ways that racist ideologies, structures, and institutions create and maintain racial inequality.

Intersectionality: Intersectionality is a framework that refers to the interconnected nature of social categorizations such as race, class, and gender, regarded as creating overlapping and interdependent systems of discrimination or disadvantage. First coined by Professor Kimberlé Crenshaw (1989), intersectionality is the acknowledgement that everyone has their own unique experiences of discrimination and oppression. The framework serves as a necessary lens through which to explore how social inequalities of race, class, gender, sexuality, age, ability, and ethnicity shape one another.

Spatial Justice: Spatial justice is a framework that entails an examination of the fair and equitable distribution in space of socially valued resources and opportunities to use them (Soja, 2010). In contemplating spatial justice, it is understood that the idea of socio-spatial relations is fundamental: that is, that space shapes social relations as much as social relations shape space.

Somebodiness: Somebodiness is a community-recognized idea rooted in African American history and expanded upon by theologians such as Howard Thurman and Dr. Martin Luther King Jr. Professor Phillip Johnson (2016) has noted that the psychological functioning of African American men is often described in negative terms and does not account for systemic racism and oppression. Therefore, the promotion of somebodiness asserts that dignity is inherent to human beings and a value to be fought for, a position which has valuable implications for Black men and boys.

References

Brown, T. (2003). Critical race theory speaks to the sociology of mental health: Mental health problems produced by racial stratification. *Journal of Health and Social Behavior, 44*(3), 292–301. Retrieved March 16, 2021, from http://www.jstor.org/stable/1519780

Butler, J. (2010). Performative acts and gender constitution: An essay in phenomenology and feminist theory. In C. McCann & S.-k. Kim (Eds.), *Feminist theory reader local and global perspectives* (pp. 419–430). Routledge.

Centers for Disease Control and Prevention. (2021). *Mental health basics*. Retrieved from https://www.cdc.gov/mentalhealth/learn/index.htm

Chavez, V. (2018). Cultural humility: Reflections and relevance for CBPR. In N. Wallerstein, B. Duran, J. Oetzel, & M. Minkler (Eds.), *Community-based participatory research for health: Advancing social and health equity* (3rd ed., pp. 357–362). Jossey-Bass.

Clark, P. A. (1998). A legacy of mistrust: African-Americans, the medical profession, and AIDS. *The Linacre Quarterly, 65*(1), 66–88. https://doi.org/10.1080/00243639.1998.11878407

Crenshaw, K. (1989). Demarginalizing the intersection of race and sex: A black feminist critique of antidiscrimination doctrine, feminist theory and antiracist politics. *University of Chicago Legal Forum, 1*, 139–167.

Culp, B. (2017). Illegitimate bodies in legitimate times: Life, liberty, and the pursuit of movement. *Quest, 69*(2), 143–156. https://doi.org/10.1080/00336297.2017.1287578

Culp, B. (2020). Thirdspace investigations: Geography, dehumanization, and seeking spatial justice in kinesiology. *Quest, 72*, 153–166. https://doi.org/10.1080/00336297.2020.1729824

DiMasso, A., Dixon, J., & Pol, E. (2011). On the contested nature of place: 'Figuera's Well', 'The Hole of Shame' and the ideological struggle over public space in Barcelona. *Journal of Environmental Psychology, 31*, 231–244. https://doi.org/10.1016/j.jenvp.2011.05.002

Du Bois, W. E. B. (1920). *Darkwater: Voices from within the veil*. Harcourt, Brace, and Howe.

Du Bois, W. E. B. (1999). *The souls of black folk. Critical edition* (H. L. Gates Jr & T. H. Oliver, Eds.). Norton. (Original work published 1903).

Fanon, F. (1967). *Black skin, white masks*. Grove.

Gara, M. A., Minsky, S., Silverstein, S. M., Miskimen, T., & Strakowski, S. M. (2019). A naturalistic study of racial disparities in diagnoses at an outpatient behavioral health clinic. *Psychiatric Services (Washington, D.C.), 70*(2), 130–134. https://doi.org/10.1176/appi.ps.201800223

Gilbert, K. L., Ray, R., Siddiqi, A., Shetty, S., Baker, E. A., Elder, K., & Griffith, D. M. (2016). Visible and invisible trends in black men's health: Pitfalls and promises for addressing racial, ethnic, and gender inequities in health. *Annual Review of Public Health, 37*, 295–311. https://doi.org/10.1146/annurev-publhealth-032315-021556

Gillborn, D. (2015). Intersectionality, critical race theory, and the primacy of racism: Race, class, gender, and disability in education. *Qualitative Inquiry, 21*(3), 277–287. https://doi.org/10.1177/1077800414557827

Greene-Moton, E., & Minkler, M. (2020). Cultural competence or cultural humility? Moving beyond the debate. *Health Promotion Practice, 21*(1), 142–145. https://doi.org/10.1177/1524839919884912

Hankerson, S. H., Suite, D., & Bailey, R. K. (2015). Treatment disparities among African American men with depression: Implications for clinical practice. *Journal of Health Care for the Poor and Underserved, 26*(1), 21–34. https://doi.org/10.1353/hpu.2015.0012

Hargrove, T. W., & Brown, T. H. (2015). A life course approach to inequality: Examining racial/ethnic differences in the relationship between early life socioeconomic conditions and adult health among men. *Ethnicity & Disease, 25*(3), 313–320. https://doi.org/10.18865/ed.25.3.313

Howard, T. C., Flennaugh, T. K., & Terry, C. L. (2012). Black males, social imagery, and the disruption of pathological identities: Implications for research and teaching. *Educational Foundations, 26*, 85–102.

Jäggi, L. J., Mezuk, B., Watkins, D. C., & Jackson, J. S. (2016). The relationship between trauma, arrest, and incarceration history among Black Americans: Findings from the national survey of American life. *Society and Mental Health, 6*(3), 187–206. https://doi.org/10.1177/2156869316641730

Johnson, P. (2016). Somebodiness and its meaning to African American men. *Journal of Counseling & Development, 94*(3), 333–343.

Jones-Eversley, S. D., Rice, J., Adedoyin, A. C., & James-Townes, L. (2020). Premature deaths of young black males in the United States. *Journal of Black Studies, 51*(3), 251–272. https://doi.org/10.1177/0021934719895999

King, C., & Gillard, S. (2019). Bringing together coproduction and community participatory research approaches: Using first person reflective narrative to explore coproduction and community involvement in mental health research. *Health Expectations: An International Journal of Public Participation in Health Care and Health Policy, 22*(4), 701–708. https://doi.org/10.1111/hex.12908

King, C., Bennett, M., Fulford, K., Clarke, S., Gillard, S., Bergqvist, A., & Richardson, J. (2021). From preproduction to coproduction: COVID-19, whiteness, and making black mental health matter. *The Lancet. Psychiatry, 8*(2), 93–95. https://doi.org/10.1016/S2215-0366(20)30458-2

Koh, A. (2017, April 3). *Placemaking when black lives matter*. Progressive City. https://www.progressivecity.net/single-post/2017/04/03/PLACEMAKING-WHEN-BLACK-LIVES-MATTER

Kumagai, A. K., & Lypson, M. L. (2009). Beyond cultural competence: Critical consciousness, social justice, and multicultural education. *Academic Medicine, 84*(6), 782–787.

Leonardo, Z. (2002). The souls of white folk: Critical pedagogy, whiteness studies, and globalization discourse. *Race, Ethnicity, and Education, 5*, 29–50.

Leonardo, Z. (2009). *Race, whiteness and education*. Routledge.

Lynch, M. E. (2018). The hidden nature of whiteness in education: Creating active allies in white teachers. *Journal of Educational Supervision, 1*, 18–31.

Mahalik, J. R., Pierre, M. R., & Wan, S. S. C. (2006). Examining racial identity and masculinity as correlates of self-esteem and psychological distress in black men. *Journal of Multicultural Counseling and Development, 34*(2), 94–104. https://doi.org/10.1002/j.2161-1912.2006.tb00030.x

Metzl, J. M. (2009). *The protest psychosis: How schizophrenia became a black disease*. Beacon Press.

Meyer, O. L., & Zane, N. (2013). The influence of race and ethnicity in clients' experiences of mental health treatment. *Journal of Community Psychology, 41*(7), 884–890.

Motley, R., & Banks, A. (2018). Black males, trauma, and mental health service use: A systematic review. *Perspectives on Social Work: The Journal of the Doctoral Students of the University of Houston Graduate School of Social Work, 14*(1), 4–19.

Murray-Garcia, J., & Tervalon, M. (2014). The concept of cultural humility. *Health Affairs, 33*(7), 1303.

Nussbaum, M. (2000). *Women and human development: The capabilities approach*. Cambridge University Press.

Painter, N. I. (2010). *The history of white people*. W. W. Norton.

Poussaint, A. F. (2002). Yes: It can be a delusional symptom of psychotic disorders. *The Western Journal of Medicine, 176*(1), 4. https://doi.org/10.1136/ewjm.176.1.4

Samson, F. L. (2018). An association between multiculturalism and psychological distress. *PLoS One, 13*(12), e0208490. https://doi.org/10.1371/journal.pone.0208490

Schwartz, R. C., & Blankenship, D. M. (2014). Racial disparities in psychotic disorder diagnosis: A review of empirical literature. *World Journal of Psychiatry, 4*(4), 133–140. https://doi.org/10.5498/wjp.v4.i4.133

Sen, A. (1999). *Commodities and capabilities* (2nd ed.). Oxford University Press.

Sen, A. (2011). *The idea of justice*. Harvard University Press.

Soja, E. W. (2010). *Seeking spatial justice*. University of Minnesota Press.

Sotero, M. (2006). A conceptual model of historical trauma: Implications for public health practice and research. *Journal of Health Disparities Research and Practice, 1*(1), 93–108.

Taylor, E., Guy-Walls, P., Wilkerson, P., & Addae, R. (2019). The historical perspectives of stereotypes on African-American males. *Journal of Human Rights and Social Work, 4*, 213–225. https://doi.org/10.1007/s41134-019-00096-y

Terrell, F., & Terrell, S. L. (1981). An inventory to measure cultural mistrust among blacks. *The Western Journal of Black Studies, 5*(3), 180–184.

Tervalon, M., & Murray-García, J. (1998). Cultural humility versus cultural competence: A critical distinction in defining physician training outcomes in multicultural education. *Journal of Health Care for the Poor and Underserved, 9*(2), 117–125. https://doi.org/10.1353/hpu.2010.0233

Thomas, A., Hammond, W. P., & Kohn-Wood, L. P. (2015). Chill, be cool man: African American men, identity, coping, and aggressive ideation. *Cultural Diversity and Ethnic Minority Psychology, 21*(3), 369–379. https://doi.org/10.1037/a0037545

Thorpe, R. J., Jr., Cobb, R., King, K., Bruce, M. A., Archibald, P., Jones, H. P., Norris, K. C., Whitfield, K. E., & Hudson, D. (2020). The association between depressive symptoms and accumulation of stress among black men in the health and retirement study. *Innovation in Aging, 4*(5), igaa047. https://doi.org/10.1093/geroni/igaa047

Tiwari, R. (2013). Ellison's invisible man: A journey from invisibility to self-definition. *Tribhuvan University Journal, 28*(1–2), 203–216. https://doi.org/10.3126/tuj.v28i1-2.26243

Toldson, I. A., Ray, K., Hatcher, S. S., & Straughn Louis, L. (2011). Examining the long-term racial disparities in health and economic conditions among hurricane Katrina survivors: Policy implications for Gulf Coast recovery. *Journal of Black Studies, 42*(3), 360–378. https://doi.org/10.1177/0021934710372893

Utsey, S. (1997). Racism and the psychological well-being of African American men. *Journal of African American Men, 3*(1), 69–87. Retrieved March 16, 2021, from http://www.jstor.org/stable/41819324

Volpe, V. V., Lee, D. B., Hoggard, L. S., & Rahal, D. (2019). Racial discrimination and acute physiological responses among black young adults: The role of racial identity. *The Journal of Adolescent Health: Official Publication of the Society for Adolescent Medicine, 64*(2), 179–185. https://doi.org/10.1016/j.jadohealth.2018.09.004

Walters, K. L., Mohammed, S. A., Evans-Campbell, T., Beltran, R. E., Chae, D. H., & Duran, B. (2011). Bodies don't just tell stories, they tell histories: Embodiment of historical trauma among American Indians and Alaska Natives. *Du Bois Review, 8*(1), 179–189.

Ward, E., & Mengesha, M. (2013). Depression in African American men: A review of what we know and where we need to go from here. *The American Journal of Orthopsychiatry, 83*(2 Pt 3), 386–397. https://doi.org/10.1111/ajop.12015

Watkins, D. C. (2012). Depression over the adult life course for African American men: Toward a framework for research and practice. *American Journal of Men's Health, 6*, 194–210. https://doi.org/10.1177/1557988311424072

Watkins, D. C., Green, B. L., Rivers, B. M., & Rowell, K. L. (2006). Depression and black men: Implications for future research. *Journal of Men's Health & Gender, 3*(3), 227–235. https://doi.org/10.1016/j.jmhg.2006.02.005

Watkins, D. C., Mitchell, J., Mouzon, D., & Hawkins, J. (2017). *Physical and mental health interventions for black men in the United States*. Retrieved from http://www.equalmeasure.org/wp-content/uploads/2017/08/Physical-and-Mental-Health-Interventions-for-Black-Men-in-the-United-States.pdf

Wells, L., & Gowda, A. (2020). *A legacy of mistrust: African Americans and the US healthcare system*. Proceedings of UCLA health (Vol. 24). Retrieved from https://proceedings.med.ucla.edu/index.php/2020/06/12/a-legacy-of-mistrust-african-americans-and-the-us-healthcare-system/

Whaley, A. L. (2001). Cultural mistrust and mental health services for African Americans: A review and meta-analysis. *The Counseling Psychologist, 29*(4), 513–531. https://doi.org/10.1177/0011000001294003

WHO. (2001). *Mental health: new understanding, new hope* (The World Health Report). World Health Organization.

Williams, D. R. (2018). Stress and the mental health of populations of color: Advancing our understanding of race-related stressors. *Journal of Health and Social Behavior, 59*(4), 466–485. https://doi.org/10.1177/0022146518814251

Yeager, K. A., & Bauer-Wu, S. (2013). Cultural humility: Essential foundation for clinical researchers. *Applied Nursing Research: ANR, 26*(4), 251–256. https://doi.org/10.1016/j.apnr.2013.06.008

Brian Culp, EdD, is a Professor and Department Chair in the Wellstar College of Health and Human Services at Kennesaw State University in Kennesaw, Georgia. He has over 20 years of experience assisting communities across the globe in their efforts to eradicate health disparities through a focus on spatiality, justice, and intergenerational physical activity programming. A recipient of several awards for his efforts, Culp has been a Fulbright Scholar in Montreal, Canada.

Part II
Black Masculinity

Chapter 4
Beyond Moving the Ball in Youth Sports: Making the Case for Mental Health for Black Youth

Vanessa Robinson-Dooley

Playing sports as a child, adolescent or teenager is often one of the highlights of our youth. It is an experience where we first learn how to get along with new people. Team sports also teach us other valuable lessons such as working with people from different backgrounds, learning to share (credit and loses), taking instruction from a stranger (coaches), and even learning to control emotions we feel with things don't go our way. We can all agree that youth sports are a valuable and important contribution to development. What is often not addressed in youth sports are the challenges that these children bring to the team or to their respective sport. Whether it be their home life, their neighborhood environment, their educational experience, and/or their mental health, youth playing sports needs to be considered from a more holistic perspective. If we want children to be able to harness their power as athletes, we must also encourage them to understand their needs as developing youth. These needs could include undiagnosed and untreated mental illness and trauma from their lived experiences. Black male youth have an even greater challenge. In a time where Black men are seen as inherently dangerous and too often the resting place of a bullet, we must begin to engage in the conversation about how we work to not only develop Black male athletes; we must also talk about what other areas these athletes need to "develop" to be able to navigate a world that uses them for their bodies but has no interest in their development as human beings, living with the same triumphs and struggles as those who do not carry the ball.

In this chapter, the focus is on making the case for intentionally integrating mental health into the youth sports system to better the overall development of Black male youth. We must move beyond them carrying the ball and focus on what athletes need to be successful in life.

V. Robinson-Dooley (✉)
School of Social Work, Simmons University, Boston, MA, USA
e-mail: vanessa.robinson-dooley@simmons.edu

© The Author(s), under exclusive license to Springer Nature Switzerland AG 2022
Y. D. Dyson et al. (eds.), *Black Men's Health*,
https://doi.org/10.1007/978-3-031-04994-1_4

Data on Black Youth and Sports

Data on youth in sports has been limited in scope and collection. The most current data reported on youth playing team/organized sports comes from the National Survey of Children's Health (https://www.childhealthdata.org) and the State of Play Report 2021 (https://www.aspenprojectplay.org). The National Survey of children reported that 56.1 % of youth reported that they have participated on a team or with sports lessons. The State of Play report provides a more detailed breakdown of the demographics of youth playing organized sports. In this report, the Aspen Institute collected data on a variety of team sports and demographics on the youth that participate in those activities. They found that between 2012 and 2020, the number of youths participating in any sport (team or individual) increased from 72.9% to 76.1% (Aspen Institute, 2021). Those reporting primarily playing team sports on a "regular basis" actually declined from 41.4% in 2012 to 37.8% in 2020. Based on the limited data from these reports, in the sample, 38.9% of Black youth participated in team sports in 2012. That number decreased slightly to 34.8% in both 2019 and 2020. Even with the limited data, these are still large numbers of Black youth playing organized sports. The numbers for participation by youth in sports for the year 2020 have to be considered in light of the COVID pandemic and the challenges that occurred for youth in school and any large gatherings, which would include sporting events.

Although there is limited data on the demographics of youth in sports, based on what is available, it is clear that there are significant numbers of youth participating in organized/team sports. There are also a significant number of young Black males participating in some aspect of sports. Any focus on the health (physical and mental) needs of Black men must also focus on their needs as youth. Impacting their health in their younger years can only serve to increase the potential for positive outcomes as adults. Youth sports could be an entry into working with this population.

Positive Youth Development and Youth Sports

The key to understanding the impact of youth sports on youth development is to recognize the important role that sports can play in the overall development of youth. Youth development can be impacted by many areas of their lives. As they age, youth will be impacted by their home life, their communities, the school they attend, social networks, social supports, and even the access and availability of health care in meeting needs. The time when youth are probably most invested in youth sports, adolescence, can be a time of significant change. Adolescence is a stage in youth development where the focus is on biological, cognitive, psychological, and social changes (Lerner, 2005). In light of the changes and what most consider a crucial time in youth development, there has been some consideration in the literature about ways in which sports and youth development intersect. Specifically, there has been discussion on how youth development should be the focus in youth sports and what areas should be considered. One of the most well-known frameworks related to this area is the Positive Youth Development (PYD) framework.

Positive Youth Development (PYD) is a framework based on the work done by the Interagency Working Group of Youth Programs (22 federal departments and youth agencies) (youth.gov, n.d.). The focus of the work of this group was to develop an approach to conducting research and practice that emphasized prevention. The idea was to move beyond the previous efforts that primarily focused on a single issue for youth and begin to consider broader ways of looking at the needs of youth and avenues for promoting positive development. The group developed the following definition of positive youth development (PYD):

> PYD is an intentional, prosocial approach that engages youth within their communities, schools, organizations, peer groups, and families in a manner that is producing and constructive; recognizes, utilizes, and enhances young people's strengths; and promotes positive outcomes for young people by providing opportunities, fostering positive relationships, and furnishing the support needed to build on their leadership strengths. (youth.gov, n.d.)

This definition and work have been used in various areas of the youth development field to begin to address the issues that youth face. The result was an understanding that one of the most effective ways to work with youth is to consider risk factors, strengths, and develop interventions and programs that would result in positive development for youth.

The literature explores the emergence of the application of Positive Youth Development used to promote successful development. Andrews and Carrano (2018) explain that the main premise of PYD is that the youth are the "resource that can be developed instead of the problem to be managed" (p. 45). These authors emphasize the framework as one viewing child development as a time of potential and on educating, understanding, and engaging in useful and productive activities (p. 45). PYD is a focus on strengths and assets, an acknowledgment that the stage of development that youth may be going through is a combination of ecology and biology. PYD posits that development is an interaction between youth and his or her context (Beck & Wiium, 2019). The contexts (i.e., home, school, neighborhood, community) represent the primary environment for youth development and can lead to the positive developmental paths that youth need (Benson, 2007).

PYD has become the overarching framework for the development of youth sports programs. Warner et al. (2019) emphasizes focusing on personal characteristics that are generally related to life skills that lead to productive lives. The authors state that this can be done with youth sports by helping youth develop "personal assets." These "personal assets" are skills and traits that assist with protection against barriers, health, and function risks that are faced by some youth (p. 2). One of the most prominent models of PYD is proposed by Lerner et al. (2005), a relational development model that focuses on the Five Cs of development competence, confidence, connection, character, and caring. The authors proposed that the characteristics of Five Cs are what the youth need for positive development. These characteristics should be the foundation for any youth programming, especially sports, to help youth thrive. Roth and Brooks-Gunn (2003) noted that the Five Cs have been linked to positive outcomes in youth development programs. Other studies have shown that participation in organized sports is associated with higher overall PYD (Andrews & Carrano, 2018). Some researchers have discovered that the amount of time a child spends participating in organized sports is associated with PYD-positive outcomes such as development of leadership skills, imitative and goal setting (Gould & Carson, 2008), higher self-esteem (Richman & Shaffer, 2000), and self-control (Fraser-Thomas et al., 2005). In considering health outcomes, researchers have noted that sports participation that focuses on PYD can impact physical fitness, reduce risky sexual behavior, and even impact suicidal ideations (Andrews & Carrano, 2018). As we consider one of the neglected areas of youth development, mental health, researchers have found that participation in youth sports can impact concentration, motivation, and emotional exploration (Larson, 1994).

If we consider the importance of encouraging positive youth development and the increasing number of youths involved in youth sports, another way that youth development can be directly impacted is if a more concerted effort is made to address mental health in youth sports.

Addressing Mental Health for Black Youth

The current times have taught us many things, but one of the most important is that Black men and Black male youth are in danger. They are in danger physically with community violence, police violence against black bodies, racism, and overall health. We know that the challenges for Black males are urgent; we also know that navigating the stage of adolescence can exacerbate the stress and concerns at that stage of their lives. Adolescence is a period of increased stress, especially for Black youth (Assari & Caldwell, 2017). While Black male youth follow the predictable development stages that we know about at this age, they may also be dealing with other factors that could include neighborhood safety, poverty or economic struggles, and educational settings that do not have their strengths or needs as a priority. Henderson et al. (2019) in their work on developing a framework focused on race-related trauma, found that Black youth are one the most vulnerable groups when thinking about health indicators. These authors discuss the many challenges that Black youth encounter which include behavioral and emotional regulation (related to trauma), being at higher risk for special education programs, school suspensions, and interaction with juvenile justice (2019). One of the starkest findings is that Black youth are at most risk for poor health outcomes. While other authors might try and make a correlation to these outcomes as a result of their neighborhood and community experiences, these health outcomes and health inequalities are more related to racism.

Henderson et al. (2019) make the best case for involving mental health earlier in the lives of Black male youth. In their literature review of investigating the challenges for Black youth and how these challenges are correlated to the racism and academics and health outcomes, they found that the areas that most informed their development of a framework for understanding race-related trauma are alienation, racial discrimination, and violence. Alienation is when the Black youth perceive differences in their learning experiences, and this is a physical and psychological disruption (2019). Alienation can also induce feelings of helplessness, powerlessness, and stress as a part of their experiences. Racial discrimination is the process of excluding or isolating a group based on race (2019). Racial discrimination can have a significant impact on Black youth's mental health as it can induce additional stress in their daily living experience. Henderson et al. (2019) discusses violence as both a physical and psychological concept. Violence impacts Black youth as both bodily harm and emotional abuse. These authors, in their development of their framework, make the case for why it is important that mental health is addressed with Black youth before there are significant outward manifestations. As with physical health and the tremendous amount of research about health disparities, the way to impact any health concern is through prevention. Another element of prevention is consistently addressing the needs of the population where they are in the context of their lives and with processes that are developed to address their specific needs.

What Can Be Done: ARMM Youth?

Youth sports have multiple ways that children participate in assessment of their skills and practice skills development. Most youth sports have organizations that plan and implement tournaments and events where youth can showcase their talents and can be seen by potential coaches and scouts. What is not present are processes or even interest in their mental health. Mental health does not necessarily mean a diagnosis that requires an extensive therapeutic treatment plan. Mental health for the purposes of this writing is defined as the overall social, emotional, and psychological well-being of the youth that could be the target of prevention, intervention, and therapeutic treatment to promote overall positive health. In some instances, the assessment might result in needs that the youth might have that are related to their family unit (food, housing, etc.) or their individual needs (physical health, mental health, education, etc.). One process that can be used as part of any sport program is "ARMM." ARMM is an acronym that stands for Assessment, Review, Manage and Monitor. ARMM (see Fig. 4.1) was developed by this author (Dr. Vanessa Robinson-Dooley), a Licensed Clinical Social Worker (LCSW) and the mother of three teenage boys whom all play travel basketball. Observation of many tournaments and games indicated a cursory need for assessment and support of Black youth in order to help foster success in their given sport, now and in the future. This author contends that if we support Black male youth early in their sporting careers, we can "ARMM" them with the tools they need to be successful athletes, students, and human beings.

ARMM is an assessment and support process that can be used with every student. The "A" in ARMM stands for Assessment. In the assessment process, athletes

Fig. 4.1 ARMM, developed by Dr. Vanessa Robinson-Dooley, LCSW

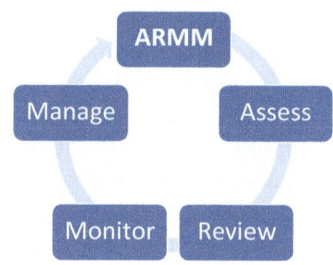

can be assessed for general daily needs (food, health, housing, etc.); they should also be assessed generally for mental health conditions. The assessment should also include an assessment of the strengths and "assets" that the young athlete currently identifies. The initial assessment can be completed by a trained case manager or human service professional. Any additional assessments for mental health needs should be done by trained mental health practitioners. There are tools that can be used as pre-assessment mental health tools to determine if more specific mental health assessment is warranted. If more specific assessments are needed, then those can be completed by trained clinicians, and a treatment plan can be created and a treatment process can begin.

The "R" in ARMM stands for Review. At this stage in the support process, the individual completing the initial assessment should create a detailed report that discusses the strengths and needs of the young athlete. The young athlete should receive a report that details the findings of the assessment. There should be a meeting with the young athlete and then a meeting with the parent or guardian. This meeting should also include any clinical assessments related to the young athlete's mental health. There should be detailed and specific recommendations intended to support the young athlete (and their family if needed). This is not a report on deficits; this is a report that builds a case for support and helping the athlete meet their goals.

The "M" in ARMM stands for Manage. Manage signifies the opportunity for the case manager to involve the athlete and his support network in their plan. Whatever goals were developed in the Review process must include action for them to be completed. In the Manage stage, the athlete and all of their support networks show their commitment to the goals set in the Review stage. Everyone explores how they will assist in managing the process and supporting the young athlete. Young athletes learn tools and explore other educational experiences that serve to build their skills and emotional development. Manage is a stage that is ongoing and an important stage in the process. The Manage stage might include some changes to the plan, or even the young athlete might change their goals. This stage should embrace flexibility and empower the young athlete not only by showing support but also by giving them the tools to meet their goals.

The last "M" in "ARMM" is Monitor. This stage is really not a defined stage but a part of the process that should be ongoing for as long as the young athlete needs support. This author contends that monitoring is needed for the life of any athlete. If we truly want to integrate mental health support in the lives of young Black athletes, we must commit to a process that requires ongoing assessment and monitoring.

Conclusion

PYD (Positive Youth Development) has been a framework discussed in the area of youth sports in recent years. Realizing that many youths will be involved in organized sports or teams at some point in their career, consideration of PYD in the planning of youth sports can assist with providing students what they might need to navigate some of the most difficult developmental stages in their lives. Based on the available statistics, we know that a significant number of Black male youth participate in youth sports. The literature also tells us that a number of Black male youth are dealing with stressors that impact their daily lives and also their ability to focus and develop in their sport of choice. It is proposed that we can also assist and support Black male youth (and truly all young athletes) by incorporating an assessment and support process like ARMM (Assessment, Review, Manage, and Monitor). The goal of ARMM is to arm students with the tools and support they need to navigate any life challenges and also provide an opportunity for any undiagnosed mental health to be treated. This can only serve to support the young Black athlete.

There is also limited evidence-based research on mental health and Black male athletes. Research determining whether intentional incorporation of mental health assessments is effective can provide the information needed to improve the process. Longitudinal studies that follow the progress of athletes when mental health is addressed and support is provided are important. Also, research on how effective youth sports really are in the development process is abstract and inconsistent.

Additional needs for youth sports include involving more social workers into the arena of youth sports. Social workers are trained professionals in human behavior and clinical work. Social workers can assist with supporting young Black athletes by assisting them with navigating their developmental process, their social and environmental needs, and mental health (clinical) needs if needed.

As we continue to involve our children in youth sports, the idea is that they are learning life skills they can use well into adulthood. Our goal should be that those life skills are those that they actually need and not those that are done by sports programs for performative purposes. If we truly want organized youth sports to be a part of the youth development process, adults must take the time to plan and "ARMM" them with what they need to succeed.

Summary
The purpose of this chapter was to explore the needs of youth athletes and explore ways that organized sports programs can assist these athletes. Positive Youth Development (PYD) is the primary framework used in any discussions of youth development in sports. PYD encourages supporting athletes in ways that will assist them with navigating the challenges of sports and the challenges of being adolescents. Black male athletes may encounter significantly more challenges than other athletes. These challenges can be the result of the impact of racism on the young Black male experience. Integrating an assessment and support process like "ARMM" into youth sports can provide an opportunity to assess, review, manage, and monitor the athlete's developmental process.

Discussion Questions

1. If you participated in youth sports in your life, what did you think were the challenges? Consider challenges that might be categorized as emotional, physical, and psychological.
2. Consider the challenges encountered by professional athletes over the years. Do you think that these challenges could have been prevented if something like the ARMM assessment and support process was introduced in youth sports?
3. What are some other ways we can assist youth through the development process while they are involved in youth posts?

Exercises

1. **Reflection Paper:** Write a brief 2- to 3-page paper reflecting on your experience in youth sports. Discuss challenges, strengths, and opportunities. (*If you did not participate in youth sports, reflect on your experience with play as a child.)
2. **Apply PYD and ARMM:** Research using library resources and news sources. Collect as much information as you can on an athlete who has dealt with trauma, mental health, violence, or legal issues. Apply the ARMM assessment and support process to the background you have collected.
3. **Infographic:** Create an infographic about the importance of mental health in youth sports.

Glossary of Terms and Concepts

PYD: Positive Youth Development, the framework used in most youth sports discussions.

ARMM: Assessment, Review, Manage, Monitor, assessment and support process.

Youth: Children ages 6–18 years participating in organized and team sports.

Youth Sports: Organized or team sports involving youth ages 6–18 years old.

Mental Health: The overall social, emotional, and psychological well-being of the youth that could be the target of prevention, intervention, and therapeutic treatment to promote overall positive health.

References

Andrews, L., & Carrano, J. (2018). Is parental participation in organized sports associated with positive youth development? *The International Journal of Sport and Society, 9*(4), 45–59. https://doi.org/10.18848/2152-7857/CGP/v09i04/45-59

Aspen Institute. (2021). *Project Play.* https://www.aspenprojectplay.org/youth-sports-facts/participation-rates

Assari, S., & Caldwell, C. H. (2017). Neighborhood safety and major depressive disorder in a national sample of Black youth. *Gender by ethnic differences. Children, 4*, 14. https://doi.org/10.3390/children4020014

Beck, M., & Wiium, N. (2019). Promoting academic achievement within a positive youth development framework. *Norsk Epidemiologi, 28*(1-2), 79–87. https://doi.org/10.5324/nje.v28i1-2.3054

Benson, P. L. (2007). Developmental assets: An overview of theory, research, and practice. In R. Silbereisen & Lerner (Eds.), *Approaches to positive youth development* (pp. 33–59). Sage Publications.

Fraser-Thomas, J. L., Côté, J., & Deakin, J. (2005). Youth sport programs: An avenue to foster positive youth development. *Physical Education and Sport Pedagogy, 10*(1), 19–40. https://doi.org/10.1080/1740898042000334890

Gould, D., & Carson, S. (2008). Life skills development through sport: Current status and future directions. *International Review of Sport and Exercise Psychology, 1*(1), 58–78.

Henderson, D. X., Walker, L., Barnes, R., Lunsford, A., Edwards, C., & Clark, C. (2019). A Framework for race-related trauma in the public education system and implications on health for Black youth. *Journal of School Health, 89*(11), 926.

Larson, R. (1994). Youth organizations, hobbies, and sports as developmental contexts. In *Adolescence in context: The interplay of family, school, peers, and work in adjustment* (pp. 46–65). Springer.

Lerner, R. M. (2005). Foreword. Urie Bronfenbrenner: Career contributions of the consummate developmental scientist. In U. Bronfenbrenner (Ed.), *Making human beings human: Bioecological perspectives on human development* (pp. ix–xxvi). Sage Publications.

Lerner, R. M., Lerner, J. V., Almerigi, J., Theokas, C., Phelps, E., Gestsdóttir, S., Naudeau, S., Jeličič, H., Alberts, A. E., Ma, L., Smith, L. M., Bobek, D. L., Richman-Raphael, D., Simpson, I., Christiansen, E. D., & von Eye, A. (2005). Positive youth development, participation in community youth development programs, and community contributions of fifth grade adolescents: Findings from the first wave of the 4-H Study of Positive Youth Development. *Journal of Early Adolescence, 25*(1), 17–71.

National Survey of Children's Health. (2019). https://www.childhealthdata.org/browse/survey/results?q=8071&r=

Richman, E. L., & Shaffer, D. R. (2000). If You Let Me Play Sports. *Psychology of Women Quarterly, 24*(2), 189–199. https://doi.org/10.1111/j.1471-6402.2000.tb00200.x

Roth, J. L., & Brooks-Gunn, J. (2003). Youth development programs: Risk, prevention and policy. *Journal of Adolescent Health, 32*, 170–182. https://doi.org/10.1016/S1054-139X(02)00421-4

Warner, M., White, G., Robinson, J., Cairney, J., & Fraser-Thomas, J. (2019). Study protocol for 2-year longitudinal study of positive youth development at an urban sport for development. *BMC Public Health, 19*(1480), 1–14. https://doi.org/10.1186/s12889-019-7843-5

Youth.gov. (n.d.). *Positive youth development.* https://youth.gov/youth-topics/positive-youth-development

Vanessa Robinson-Dooley, LCSW, CNP received her BA in Political Science from Spelman College in Atlanta, Georgia. She also holds a Master of Public Administration (MPA) from Drake University, and Master (MSW) and Doctor of Social Work from The University of Georgia. She is a Licensed Clinical Social Worker in the state of Georgia. Her direct practice (therapist) experience includes individual and family therapy, group work, and assessments. She has also worked in the area of domestic violence, program development, and community organizing. Dr. Robinson-Dooley's research focus includes factors surrounding chronic diseases and behavioral health in African American men, and promoting cultural competency in education and practice. She is Co-PI on a $700,000 NIH grant with two colleagues from Kennesaw State University in Kennesaw, Georgia, studying self-management of chronic disease and behavioral health for Black men and developing a peer-led curriculum. Dr. Robinson-Dooley is teaching courses on "teaching" and is an advocate of UDL (Universal Design for Learning) principles and technology use in the classroom. She has published in multiple journals and presented nationally on various topics related to her teaching and research.

Chapter 5
The Psychological Colonization of Black Masculinity: Decolonizing Mainstream Psychology for White Allies Working in Mental Health with Black Men

Hans Skott-Myhre and Kathleen Skott-Myhre

We find ourselves in an awkward position. We are two privileged, white academics who are clearly the beneficiaries of a colonial system we are about to critique. Perhaps even more problematically, we are proposing to critique white colonial logic within a book about the health of Black men that takes a "strength-based approach through a social justice lens." There are several inherent contradictions in our positioning within such a book. In the first place, what business do we have as white academics to write on an issue perhaps best addressed by the Black community itself? Second, what could we have to offer to Black men who are the focus of the book? After all, one of us is a white woman, and the other is male, but certainly not Black. Of course, some of the criteria for inclusion in the book fit. As clinicians, we have been trained in, practiced, and taught, an approach to working with people from a strength-based perspective. Further, we have a long-standing investment in social justice as a lens. However, even that kind of background may not give us sufficient pass as "good white people" who have the right to speak here.

So, what is our claim to be in this book? Perhaps, the audiences we want to address here are people precisely like us who will read this book. White clinicians who are working in mental health intending to be helpful to Black men. We want to talk to *our* people because we believe that as white academics involved in the "helping professions," we have accountability to be responsive to the harm white professionals have done through "helping."

Let's begin here. We would argue that the mental health issues attributed to Black men can be directly correlated to living in a society that is toxic to them at every

H. Skott-Myhre (✉)
Department of Social Work and Human Services, Kennesaw State University,
Kennesaw, GA, USA
e-mail: hskottmy@kennesaw.edu

K. Skott-Myhre
Psychology Program, University of West Georgia, Carrollton, GA, USA

Y. D. Dyson et al. (eds.), *Black Men's Health*,
https://doi.org/10.1007/978-3-031-04994-1_5

57

level. We would further propose that until that simple realization is evident to every white "helping" professional they encounter, each encounter is an inevitable site of re-traumatization. Simply put, before we can even begin a conversation about the psychological or psychiatric coordinates of Black men's mental health, we need to fully address the forces of colonization and racism that shape the society in which their bodies and minds are situated.

In a way, we suggest that white "helping" professionals, in particular, cannot help but be complicit in practices that perpetuate the same system that produces the ongoing trauma experienced by Black men on a daily basis. We are not suggesting that white "helping" professionals cannot work with Black men. Instead, we are unequivocally stating that white clinicians and mental health workers need to *unontologize* themselves before such work is engaged.

We borrow the term unontologize from McKenzie (2020), who argues that the very core of white identity is saturated with the logics of colonialism. White subjectivity is inherently disposed toward the colonization of the "other." This particular logic of colonization goes beyond the discourses of white privilege. We would suggest that white privilege is an effect that points to a more foundational cause. That cause is found in the truth claims of the European colonial project. As a set of truth claims, white privilege is epistemological or how we make sense of the world in which we live. It is an implied explanation that is so ingrained as to be nearly invisible. It is a functioning linguistic code that plays itself out in an almost infinite set of micro-interactions on a daily basis. As white mental health workers and clinicians, our privilege is implied in the way we enter a room, position ourselves in "our" office, hold a clipboard, render a diagnosis, give a look, speak with an authoritarian tone of voice, or offer a compassionate word laced with the superiority of assumed safety. The list is long and exceedingly subtle and constitutes the language of white supremacy that can pass unnoticed because it is implied rather than overtly spoken. It is epistemological in that it is the expression of how we know the world and what is true. Also, regrettably, whether we can bring it into consciousness or not, to be nominally white in the early part of the twenty-first century still carries the truth of colonial rule as an actuality, not as an historical artifact.

Lacan (2006) tells us that our unconscious is structured like a language, and it is his student Guattari (2011) who tells us that we get the unconscious we deserve. The unconscious referenced here is both individual and collective. Not collective in the sense of the Jungian collective unconscious with its highly problematic universalist archetypes but collective in the sense of a commonly derived social set of templates that shape our conscious understanding of the world and our place in it. This collective unconscious is comprised and re-comprised in every historical period out of the drives to control and dominate, as well as the resultant traumas and drives toward liberation. In this regard, the unconscious created in the process of colonization produces ways of making sense that deeply inflect the construction of our subjectivity. Lacan (2006) refers to these as signifiers, and the most powerful signifier for colonization is whiteness.

Whiteness is what Lacan referred to as a master signifier or a signifier that points only to itself. In other words, whiteness operates at an unconscious level as the central defining term to which all other terms of social investment must return. To be white is a social signifier that defines all social relationships within global capitalism. To work toward being anti-racist is to refuse whiteness this role in our society. Unfortunately, most anti-racist work is primarily done at the level of conscious discourse as an intentional set of social policies or personal reidentification.

Of course, those of us who work in mental health know that conscious attempts to reformulate our behavior simply by raising our awareness often founder on the hidden rocks of our unconscious desires. To a large degree, the effects of our unconscious desires are why consciousness-raising anti-racist training doesn't work (Bergner, 2020). Conscious awareness doesn't have a lasting impact on behavior. Our unconscious has a million subtle ways to undo and derail our best conscious intentions.

It is vital to be clear that whiteness is a collective delusion even to begin to address the latent racism embedded in the social unconscious of the inheritors of colonial logic. This delusion is an expression of paranoiac thinking reinforced through fascist modes of social organization. Whiteness as an expression of colonial logic is a paranoid delusion that can only be sustained through continual modulations of the "truth." That is to say, whiteness as a master signifier can only retain its centrality through constant manipulation of social descriptions that simultaneously obscure its force while distributing its logic at every level of society. Like all paranoid delusions, all information about the world must be made to fit within the logic of white supremacy. However, to avoid any significant challenge to this system of delusion, the central role that colonial logic plays in the continuance of the current system of rule must be hidden from view. We can have endless discussions and social policy initiatives that address race and racism, white privilege, reparations for slavery, and so on, as long as the colonial logic that keeps producing new forms of slavery and "othering" are not overthrown.

The effect of the paranoiac delusion of colonial logic operates at both the level of social discourse and at the material level in producing taxonomies, hierarchies, geographical mappings of nations and continents, and the distribution of bodies across territories. It also operates as an arbiter of geographies of subjectivity.

Our very personal subjective geography is shaped into bodies, minds, and affects appropriate to the utilitarian appropriative desire of settler-colonial capitalism. It is not just our ways of knowing that are reshaped and then reshaped again. The linguistic descriptors of our "self" are constantly undergoing revision and modulation. Our epistemology is an open cipher to be filled by whatever variables the appropriative machine of capitalism deems worth disseminating. While descriptors are a significant component of subjectification, at some level, it is simply the window dressing of the deeper reconfiguration of our ontological self.

Our ontological self both precedes and is antecedent to language. Ontologically, we are quite simply the body and its acts. We are thoroughly material, and the colonial project has historically been deeply invested in reshaping our corporeal existence so that we come to believe that our bodies, neurological responses, and ecological coevolutionary actions are saturated with capitalist logic. It is the colonial imperative that we don't just belong to capitalism, but we are *literally* capitalism. Our very beingness is entangled and conscripted into modes of living that steal us from ourselves and produce us as living addendums to the logic of the ruling system. This entanglement is why we must unontologize ourselves before we can even begin to have a meaningful conversation about mental health. As it stands, we, as white clinicians and mental health professionals, are anything but mentally healthy. In fact, the deeper we are ensnared by colonial/capitalist logic, the more we disseminate madness and suffering in our very efforts to be helpful. Like a silent carrier of disease, we unwittingly spread a viral epidemic of erasure that promotes the colonial project of appropriation, exploitation, and evisceration of Black male identity.

Frantz Fanon (2008) articulates the dilemma of colonial erasure concerning the construction of Black subjectivity under conditions of colonial rule. He points out how any originary sense of Black identity is reconfigured in such a way as to remove any vestige of independence from the definitions of whiteness as a master signifier. As he states in *Black Skin, White Masks*, "colonialism is not satisfied merely with holding a people in its grip and emptying the native's brain of all form and content. By a kind of perverted logic, it turns to the past of the oppressed people, and distorts, disfigures, and destroys it" (Fanon, 2008, p. 210).

As we have noted above, the colonial project reconfigures the topography of those subject to its rule until there is nothing recognizable but nostalgia. The ongoing process of colonization in the twenty-first century raises subject-scaping to a form of high perversity in brutally commodifying all efforts to recuperate and revitalize Black masculinity as a defense against complete erasure. In his work on Black masculinity, Tommy Curry (2017) points to historical accounts of Black male trauma from slavery forward that are notably absent from academic and popular narratives about race in North America. When Black male trauma is accounted for, it is almost always an individualized and a historical psychological explanation of pathology (Ginwright, 2018).

In a way, we might say that the colonial project is making every effort to erase the actuality of Black male trauma and replace it with a cipher to turn the actual material conditions of Black masculine life into pure representation or a symbol that can be appropriated and marketed. In turning the lived experience of Black men into a media spectacle of danger and violence, twenty-first-century capitalism turns living Black male bodies into ghosts that haunt society but have a mythological quality of unreality at the same time.

This is the complex social algebra that white clinicians and mental health workers engage when they attempt to be helpful to Black men who are suffering under current social conditions. Of course, colonization does not stop with reconfiguring the subjectivity of the marginalized and oppressed. White subjects must also be transformed into vehicles for colonial transmission. Their social coordinates concerning the "other" must be carefully calibrated so as to allow the current social system to perpetuate itself while appearing to fight for justice for all.

Edward Said (1985) speaks to the production of the colonizer as a highly disciplined response to the colonized. The colonizer as a social subject must represent the values, habits, and beliefs of the dominant system of rule in a deeply reflexive manner. The nuances of appropriate thought, speech, glance, and behavior must convey the hierarchy of colonization in every interaction. Even the most well-intentioned and benevolent set of interactions must distinguish the colonizer from the colonized. This distinction of the colonizer from the colonized is a deep level of multigenerational social induction that operates at the subtlest levels. This acculturated level of interaction is often not apparent to the colonizer but is always evident to the colonized, who must read it to survive.

It is important to note that this is what Brennan terms a "psychotic fantasy" that conceives the colonizer "as the origin cause and end of knowledge" (cited in Seshadri-Crooks, 2000, p. 4). It is the colonizer's perspective that will overcode any other counter-understanding or explanation of the world. In fact, alternative narratives are branded fantasy. Any knowledge the colonized has of themselves will be repressed through overt attempts at re-education and more subtle means of disqualification or elision.

Colonial modes of disqualification are what underlies Spivak's question (2016); can the subaltern speak? She argues that anything said by subaltern (in our case, Black male) groups will by necessity be translated into the vernacular of colonization. It will never be read on its own terms. In that sense, Spivak argues that the speech of the colonized is foreclosed. This ability to deny any knowledge the colonial other has of themselves allows for the colonizer to construct a purely imaginary projection of truly psychotic proportions that can come to stand in for the material actuality of genocidal trauma. As Fanon (2008) put it:

> there is no longer any doubt that the true "Other" for the white man is and remains the black man, and vice versa. For the white man, however, "the Other" is perceived as a bodily image, absolutely as the nonego, i.e., the unidentifiable, the unassimilable. (p. 139)

That is to say that for the colonizer, Black men as the colonial other are incomprehensible and without an independent identity. Although they may be physically directly in front of the white clinician and speaking, they cannot be seen or heard. Anything presented physically, psychologically, phenomenologically, historically, spiritually, or emotionally will be, at best, misread and at worst made incomprehensible to the speaker through translation. Nathaniel Harrington (Ovitt, 2020) speaks to this concerning the mental health response to the trauma of the George Floyd murder and the traumatic effect on Black men. He reminds us that even when Black people seek psychotherapy, they often encounter white clinicians who fail to comprehend that being Black in America is a source of persistent and powerful stress. The experience of this kind of stress is unique and can't really be interpelated into traditional mental health frameworks. Harrington notes that research suggests that the pain of being Black in America is frequently treated by White clinicians with subtle degrees of dismissiveness and/or indifference. The implication being that this kind of pain is of a lesser degree. Also, it is here that we come to the heart of the matter.

At the core of mental health work is human suffering. To the degree that suffering is acknowledged in its complexity and depth, there is some chance to alleviate the pain. To the degree suffering is obscured or treated with subtle indifference, the encounter with mental health will only perpetuate and very possibly amplify the degree of suffering experienced by Black men seeking assistance. In his letter to his son, Ta-Nehisi Coates (2020) describes the way that racism impacts Black men at a visceral level. He insists that the damage done to the body in the way that it impacts the ability to think, to breathe, to feel causes massive physical trauma to the body and mind. He tells his sone that all the ways we try to talk about racism hides the powerful and immutable physical trauma from view. He admonishes his son to never avoid this. Yet, we as white clinicians and mental health workers do look away with regularity, and we use phrasing to obscure racism. In the practice arena of mental health, we would argue that the obscuring mechanism is the machine at the very heart of the field, Eurocentric mainstream psychology.

Ian Parker (2007) has written powerfully about the collusion between mainstream psychology and capitalism/colonialism. He argues that the central precepts of mainstream psychology have worked seamlessly to obscure the social etiology of human suffering. From its inception, mainstream psychology has served as a tool for colonizing our sense of who we are and why we experience pain and trauma. Mainstream psychology focuses on the individual's experience as the source of pathology and has trained the clinician to see individual pathology as the primary focus of their work. The primary focus in mainstream psychology, with its colonial taxonomies of diagnosis, is on what has gone wrong with this individual and how we return them to functioning seamlessly within the machinery of exploitation and appropriation that is the ongoing colonial/capitalist project. The concept of historical collective trauma is nowhere to be found in the dominant vernacular of mainstream psychology. Also, it is mainstream psychology that has colonized the clinical practices of social work and the practices of other mental health practitioners.

The individualizing orientation of mainstream psychology, focusing on faulty neurology and biological malfunction, is the most obvious iteration of a long history of racism. Key concepts and ideas that drive the practices and training of clinicians and mental health workers are riddled with white supremacist histories. If these ideas were statues, the same clinicians who inherited these ideas and practices without serious reflection would insist on their removal. For example, the founders of statistical analysis that so profoundly influences psychological research and training were well-known eugenicists and racists, including Sir Francis Galton, Karl Pearson, and Sir Ronald A. Fischer. Similarly, developmental psychologist G. Stanley Hall was also a eugenicist. Paul Popenoe, the founder of American marriage counseling, argued that the amount of white blood one has is correlated with intelligence. In 1916, Lewis Madison Terman, the developer of the Stanford-Binet IQ test and president of the American Psychological Association, asserted that Black people have a dullness that is attributable to their race, and their children should be put in special classes where they can learn concrete skills because abstraction is beyond their abilities (Williams, 2020).

In a statement released in January of 2021, the American Psychiatric Association (2021) issued an apology to Black, Indigenous, and People of Color (BIPOC) for structural racism in psychiatry. It read in part:

Since the APA's inception, practitioners have at times subjected persons of African descent and Indigenous people who suffered from mental illness to abusive treatment, experimentation, victimization in the name of "scientific evidence," along with racialized theories that attempted to confirm their deficit status. Similar race-based discrepancies in care also exist in medical practice today as evidenced by the variations in schizophrenia diagnosis between white and BIPOC patients, for instance. These appalling past actions, as well as their harmful effects, are ingrained in the structure of psychiatric practice and continue to harm BIPOC psychological well-being even today. Unfortunately, the APA has historically remained silent on these issues. As the leading American organization in psychiatric care, the APA recognizes that this inaction has contributed to perpetuation of structural racism that has adversely impacted not just its own BIPOC members, but also psychiatric patients across America. (para 2)

While apologies such as this by dominant groups have a confirmatory aspect that, at a minimum, lets subjugated and oppressed groups know that they are not "crazy," the apology itself does not stop the colonial practices of the dominant group. That requires a complete repudiation of all aspects of the mental health system that is so deeply colonized by psychiatry and psychology. For white clinicians and mental health workers, we need to recognize that our training and research are deeply and unconsciously founded in this system of structural racism. We need to acknowledge that the use of statistical tools, diagnostic manuals, clinical assessments, IQ tests, personality tests, developmental frameworks, and psychiatric/psychological definitions of trauma are derived from what the APA itself has identified as a system premised in structural racism. We also must understand that psychiatry/psychology as a colonizing tool produces us as colonizers who disseminate colonial practices to the Black men we encounter in our work. As the colonizer, we encourage Black men to adopt the language of diagnosis rooted in structural racism that subtly shapes their self-perception. Of course, we can say that we are using a "strength-based" perspective, but how much of that outlook is still influenced by diagnosis and notions of individualized trauma? To what end are we utilizing strength-based technologies? Is it to the purpose of successfully colonizing our Black male clients into accepting the idea that their success is to be found in assimilation?

We have suggested in this chapter that it is essential to our work, as white allies working with Black men in a mental health context, that we refuse our role in the ongoing colonial/capitalist project. We have suggested that to refuse such a role requires a process of deep self-reflection through which we unontologize ourselves as settler-colonists. We have argued that it is imperative that we simultaneously acknowledge our whiteness and its attendant privilege while refusing it every time it arises within ourselves. To undo our colonial subjectivity is not a process with a conclusion; it is a day at a time set of accountabilities. Further, we would contend that our participation in the institutions of psychology and psychiatry (and clinical social work by association) are profoundly problematic and can substantively interfere with our capacity to engage with Black male suffering authentically. We insist that it is necessary to dismantle the mechanisms of structural racism in our work, such as diagnostic and developmental frameworks and psychological assessments of intelligence and psychopathology.

We recognize that there are alternative models of care coming into practice, such as critical psychology, liberation psychology, radical social work, narrative therapy, just therapy, and progressive human services, among others. We deliberately have not engaged these approaches here because we would contend that until we engage the primary work of unontologizing ourselves, such practices can be unwittingly turned back into mechanisms for denial and colonization.

At the end of the day, we would call for white allies to take the ongoing trauma of being Black and male in contemporary society very seriously. It is to that experience that we are accountable as ongoing progenitors of that trauma. We are not interested in promoting guilt or shame about our involvement in the process of violence and continued attempts at genocide. However, we are calling for profound levels of ongoing accountability. As clinicians whose work is dedicated to, at a minimum, *do no harm*, it is the least we can do.

Summary
In this chapter, we have argued that imposing traditional psychological frameworks on Black masculinity is an inherently colonial project that uses Eurocentric psychology as the preferred template for diagnosing and treating suffering and misery in Black men. To produce a genuinely responsive system of mental health care to the needs of Black men requires that providers stop centering Black masculinity around Eurocentric psychological ideas and systems of diagnosis and treatment. For white allies, the ability to think outside the colonial frameworks of traditional psychology is imperative to any successful cross-cultural collaboration.

Discussion Questions
1. What is the relationship between colonization, whiteness, and clinical practice with Black men?
2. Given psychology/psychiatry's history and contemporary practices of structural racism, are psychology/psychiatry still appropriate for working with Black men?
3. The chapter calls for deep reflection on white clinician's role as colonizers. What would that look like to you?

Exercises
1. Give three examples of how you might rethink the use of diagnosis as a colonial process when working with Black men.
2. Pay particular attention to how you feel when working with Black men because much of our colonial instincts operate unconsciously outside of our rational perceptions. Keep a daily journal noting the times that you are inducted into colonial thinking as a therapist, psychologist, or social worker.
3. Complete an intersectional inventory of yourself identifying your position related to class, gender, race, and sexuality. Reflect on the levels of privilege you have that are based on your inventory. Write down how you think this might impact how you see and are seen by your clients.
4. In this chapter, we have argued that the mental health field is heavily influenced by psychiatry and psychology. We have also made the case that psychiatry and

psychology are inherently colonial structures that historically have had negative impacts on Black men. How do you reconcile this with a professional identity as a mental health clinician? How might you think about your professional identity outside of these colonial structures?

Glossary of Terms and Concepts

Cipher: We mean cipher in its sense of a fictional character who is a blank slate.

Colonial/colonization/colonial logic: Colonial refers to the European land theft and enslavement project that we would argue is ongoing. We would note that we are writing from a Settler State (the United States) context where the colonizers still maintain political and economic dominance. Colonization refers to the processes of the colonial project, which includes land theft and enslavement and efforts at cultural erasure and physical genocide, which we would argue are still being used today, albeit in evolving new forms. Colonial logic refers to the philosophical conceptual frameworks used to justify colonization which we would argue are still very active in the twenty-first century.

Colonizer/colonized/subaltern: Colonizer refers to those subjects inducted in acting on behalf of the colonial project consciously or unconsciously. Colonized refers to those subject to colonial rule. Spivak and Riach (2016) defines subaltern as any group that must appeal to a dominant group for basic survival needs. We would argue that all these categories are very active in the twenty-first-century global economy.

Discourse: We are using the term as defined by Foucault (1980) as ways of knowing that become common social practice. Such common ways of speaking about the world are full of power relations rooted in who can speak and what can be said to be true.

Epistemology: The study of how we know what we know. In our context, it is a system of meaning-making that shapes what we know and how we know it.

Fascist: We follow Deleuze and Guattari (1987), who define fascism as any system that forecloses difference. That is a system that insists on its logic alone and no other logic. Also, see Foucault's guide to Ant-Fascist Living (1987).

Ideology: A system of belief which we would argue, following Marx and Engels (1970), is generally premised in the logic of the ruling class.

Signifier/master signifier: Signifier we define following Lacan (2006) as the basic units of language used to create a social world. The master signifier is a signifier that turns all other signifiers to itself to make meaning.

Subaltern: Following Spivak and Riach (2016), we would define this as a subjugated group dependent upon a dominant group for the things they need to survive.

Subjectivity/subjectification: We define subjectivity as the intrinsic qualities of being a subject, i.e., thoughts, perceptions, and feelings. Subjectification is the social process of shaping subjectivity.

Unontologize/ontology: We use the following McKenzie (2020) to mean the process of undoing a state of being created through a social process. In our case, that process is colonization. Ontology is the study of how we know what is or what is being and becoming.

References

American Psychiatric Association. (2021). APA's apology to Black, Indigenous and People of Color for its support of structural racism in psychiatry. *APA Newsroom*. https://www.psychiatry.org/newsroom/apa-apology-for-its-support-of-structural-racism-in-psychiatry

Bergner, D. (2020). 'White fragility' is everywhere: But does antiracism training work? *New York Times*. https://www.nytimes.com/2020/07/15/magazine/white-fragility-robin-diangelo.html?action=click&module=Well&pgtype=Homepage&section=The%20New%20York%20Times%20Magazine

Coates, T.-N. (2020). Letter to my son. *The Atlantic*. https://www.theatlantic.com/politics/archive/2015/07/tanehisi-coates-between-the-world-and-me/397619/

Curry, T. J. (2017). *The man-not: Race: Class, genre, and the dilemmas of Black manhood*. Temple University Press.

Deleuze, G., & Guattari, F. (1987). *A thousand plateaus: Capitalism and schizophrenia*. University of Minnesota Press.

Fanon, F. (2008). *Black skin, white masks*. Grove Press.

Foucault, M. (1980). *Power/knowledge: Selected interviews and other writings, 1972–1977*. Vintage.

Foucault, M. (1987). Preface: Guide to anti-fascist living. In G. Deleuze & F. Guattari (Eds.), *A thousand plateaus: Capitalism and schizophrenia* (B. Massumi, Trans.). University of Minnesota.

Ginwright, S. (2018). The future of healing: Shifting from trauma informed care to healing centered engagement. *Occasional Paper, 25*.

Guattari, F. (2011). *The machinic unconscious*. MIT Press.

Lacan, J. (2006). *Ecrits: The first complete edition in English*. WW Norton & Company.

Marx, K., & Engels, F. (1970). *The German ideology* (Vol. 1). International Publishers Co.

McKenzie, K. (2020). *Unsettlering white settler child and youth care pedagogy and practice: Discourses on working in colonial violence and racism*.

Ovitt, N. (2020). "A complicated pain": Systemic racism's impact on Black Americans' mental health. *Michigan Radio*. https://www.michiganradio.org/post/complicated-pain-systemic-racism-s-impact-black-americans-mental-health

Parker, I. (2007). *Revolution in psychology: Alienation to emancipation*. Pluto Press.

Said, E. (1985). *Orientalism: Western representations of the orient [1978]*. Penguin.

Seshadri-Crooks, K. (2000). *Desiring whiteness: A Lacanian analysis of race*. Psychology Press.

Spivak, G. C., & Riach, G. (2016). *Can the subaltern speak?* (p. 254). Macat International Limited.

Williams, M. T. (2020). Psychology's hidden history: Racist roots and poison fruits. *Psychology Today*.

Hans Skott-Myhre, PhD, is a professor in the Department of Social Work and Human Services at Kennesaw State University in Kennesaw, Georgia. He is the author of *Youth Subcultures as Creative Force: Creating New Spaces for Radical Youth Work* (University of Toronto Press), co-author of *Habitus of the Hood* (The University of Chicago Press), co-editor of *With Children and Youth* (Wilfrid Laurier University Press) and *Youth Work, Early Education and Psychology: Liminal Encounters* (Palgrave Macmillan), as well as co-editor of *Art as Revolt: Thinking Politics Through Immanent Aesthetics* (McGill-Queen's University Press). Most recently he is the author of *Post-Capitalist Subjectivity in Literature and Anti-Psychiatry: Reconceptualizing the Self Beyond Capitalism* (Routledge). He has published multiple articles, reviews and book chapters.

Kathleen Skott-Myhre, PsyD, is Professor of Psychology at the University of West Georgia. She is the author of *Feminist Spirituality under Capitalism: Witches, Fairies and Nomads* (Routledge) as well as the co-author of *Writing the Family: Women, Auto-ethnography, and Family Work* (Sense Publishers). She is co-editor with V. Pacini-Ketchabaw and H.A. Skott-Myhre of *Youth Work, Early Education and Psychology: Liminal Encounters* (Palgrave Macmillan). She has published multiple articles, reviews and book chapters.

Chapter 6
Black Masculinity Remixed

Troy Harden and John Zeigler

Introduction

The murder of George Floyd by police officer Derek Chauvin sparked an already existing #BlackLivesMatter movement toward a new reckoning of racial identity and relations. At a cultural, institutional, and interpersonal level, questions associated with the definitions of systemic racism and racial bias are being asked and discussed at all levels of social interaction. Included within these discussions is the understanding of how systemic racism has impacted Black[1] men, both in the United States and throughout the African diaspora. However, few of these explore the complexity of Black masculinity, and some scholars speak to the importance or non-essentialist notions of Blackness. This chapter will discuss some of this range and bring forth how programs are shaped and notions of Black male identity are constructed for the sake of social programs. In highlighting three diverse efforts in an urban city, the chapter challenges assumptions on Black males. The authors invite those who work with Black men and boys to "remix" old tropes of masculinity to offer a twenty-first century progression toward social, political, and economic goals. Via exploring work done with three programs in the city of Chicago that target a range of Black men and boys, this chapter will unpack the assumptions, attitudes,

---

[1] The authors use the terms "Black" and "African American" interchangeably in this text.

T. Harden (✉)
Department of Sociology, Texas A & M University, College Station, TX, USA
e-mail: tharden@tamu.edu

J. Zeigler
Egan Office of Neighborhood and School Partnerships, DePaul University, Chicago, IL, USA
e-mail: jzeigler@depaul.edu

Y. D. Dyson et al. (eds.), *Black Men's Health*,
https://doi.org/10.1007/978-3-031-04994-1_6

beliefs, programming efforts, and strengths and difficulties of creating programs that are homogenous without respect for both the common tropes of Black masculinity and the hidden aspects of their experiences. Implications for social workers and social service providers will be discussed.

"At Risk": Masculinity, Black Men, and Boys in Social Science Research

Masculinity is a social descriptor that travels, with meaning varying by region, clan, family, and country. In Western culture, this descriptor is generally defined as gendered based on traditional notions of masculinity. However, gender roles have become complex as one can be identified as cis female, transgender, bigender, pangender, transsexual, androgynous, and so forth. For those identified as Black men and boys, this is further complicated by the popular culture depiction of the black masculine body as criminal, angry, and incapacitated.

Jackson and Elmore (2017) detail what they consider as four main forms of masculinity:

1. Dominant or hegemonic form of masculinity is defined as the idea of "real manhood" that has developed in a particular culture in order for men to have power over women and other men.
2. The subordinate form of masculinity is defined as the male behavior that threatens the legitimacy of hegemonic masculinity. This form of masculinity is exemplified by men who identify as homosexual or present as effeminate.
3. The complicit form of masculinity is defined as the man's dominant position in the gender order which allows for the "patriarchal payoff." This form of masculinity benefits from the social dominance of men.
4. The last form of masculinity is marginalization. This form of masculinity is defined as the adaptation of masculinities to the issues of race and class. This form of masculinity best describes Black masculinity where the perceived gender behavior of the male is determined not just by his sex but also by his race.

Arguably, toxic masculinity could also be considered a form that may be reflective of both hegemonic and complicit masculinity, as it invokes the belief that some people's idea of "manliness" perpetuates domination, homophobia, misogynistic tendencies, and aggression, and can be the "default" masculinity for many men.

Although masculinity has been explored in the literature, there are only recent studies that have begun to unpack how Black men perform masculinity, and the diverse ways that Black men demonstrate identity in public and private spheres. This performance of masculinity borrows from the larger social construct of masculinity but can diverge in individual ways (Bowleg et al., 2017; Dean, 2013; Griffith et al., 2012). Much of the literature examines Black men at-risk, and their behavior within systems, or at the communal and interpersonal level. Because the research is often done by psychologists, social workers, education researchers, and sociologists, at both an epistemological and theoretical level, they are centered on either pathology or help-seeking behaviors designed to understand the best way to intervene at the human service, health, or educational level and limit the framing of multiple intersecting identities that converge with gender (Bowleg et al., 2017; Young, 2017). Although important, and critical in addressing the many disparities that exist between other races and ethnicities and Black men, the framing of Black men in need of services positions much of the literature to emphasize the problem areas at best or focus on identity as a particular construct toward a detrimental behavior in need of intervention (Unnever & Chouhy, 2020).

The seminal text "Cool Pose" provides an example here. *Cool Pose: The Dilemmas of Black Manhood* (Majors & Billson, 1992) offered a view into coping for Black men, grounding behavior that may seem guarded as "protective," noting Black masculinity particularly within the urban context. However, Unnever and Chouhy (2020), in a national study of Black and white masculinity, noted that cool pose may be a normative response to the aggression they face, suggesting that research should account for what may be a normal response to oppression. Although important in guiding the arch of research that can place the onus not on Black men to adhere to US culture norms, the danger is that the framing decides that what is protective can be worked through as opposed to supported and enhanced. The theoretical construct of intersectionality as it is applied to Black boys and men (masculinity) can perhaps clear a picture into understanding social context, identity, and social behaviors toward a more comprehensive view of Black men and boys.

Intersectionality is the study of how overlapping social identities intersect and their related systems of oppressive institutions (homophobia, racism, transphobia, xenophobia, classism, etc.) are interrelated and can't be assessed separately from one another. Intersectionality theory proposes that one should think that the trait of a person is inextricably linked with all the other traits or elements to entirely recognize a person's identity and shared and lived experiences with others of comparable social identities (Crenshaw, 1989). Rooted in Black feminism and critical race theory (CRT), intersectionality is an analytic tool and disposition. Kimberlé Crenshaw introduced the term in her landmark essay "Demarginalizing the Intersection of Race and Sex: A Black Feminist Critique of Antidiscrimination Doctrine, Feminist Theory and Antiracist Politics." The essay argues that a black woman's experience cannot be understood in separate terms of being a woman and black. Crenshaw maintains that the interaction between the two identities frequently reinforce each other. Crenshaw's writing opened up further scholarship and activism concerning intersectionality and its meaning but has mostly been regulated to feminist, queer, or gender studies. Social work has benefited from this theoretical construct, as cultural proficiency is a clear value for many social workers, thus creating the opportunity to explore how intersectionality impacts participants. Intersectionality and Black masculinity mostly has focused upon the gay, bisexual, trans, and queer (GBTQ) communities, and little has been done to explore core identity markers as class, nationality and citizenship status, ability, or military status, to name a few, as these are intersecting identities that impact Black masculinity. By framing masculinity with the intersectionality approach, the field can view these identities not as problem areas but as core parts of identity that should not be marginalized in treating but add to the complexity of approaches in addressing Black men and boys. As well, because of its pro-feminist and gendered application, it can be highlight how elements of hegemonic masculinity fuse into patriarchy and oppression demonstrated by Black men, as well as how Black men are also victims of oppression in a racist society. Some scholars and activists, in discussing how education creates a school-to-prison pipeline for African American youth, posed the problem with viewing Black men and boys "at-risk" (Swadener, 1995; Fine, 1990). Social services in particular, similar to education, but arguably more demonstrative with the labels of at-risk, are guilty of this, as every stage of involvement for Black males has to be clear on "risk" level in order to provide services, including, but not limited to, program recruitment, intake, assessment, intervention design, referral, and evaluation. Addressing males as risky may enhance an already existing bias, which complicates the process for true authentic interventions to take place. An area to explore how Black men and boys have been viewed positively and take into account social factors that lead to social change may be exploring social movements and their subsequent involvement in community change.

Social Movements and Black Masculinity

Since the onset of Africans upon North American soil, there has been resistance to the oppression they faced (Engle, 2018). There is large agreement that this has taken place at both the individual level and group level. On an individual level, those enslaved have sought to purchase their freedom, ran away from plantations, educated themselves both formally and informally, and sought to position themselves for greater opportunity when available. At a group level, slave insurrections, abolishment movements, the underground railroad, and court battles have all been documented as measures that enslaved and free Blacks employed to undermine slavery (Graves Holmes, 1994). This has extended from the Reconstruction period through the Civil Rights movement: Black men and boys, and Black women and girls both besides them and leading efforts, have fought for equality and equity at the social and economic level. Slave narratives helped capture the complex identity formation that took place for those under the worst conditions. Du Bois (1903/1999), in his seminal work, captured this mixed identity in his seminal work "Souls of Black Folks," discussing the double consciousness that Black people in the United States feel, exemplified in both their internal identity and the identity projected upon them by the white gaze.

Much has been written about how key Black men who figured in the intellectual and social framing of many of these movements identified and used theoretical assumptions concerning Black progress toward their efforts. Many of these figures' differences have also been written about including such hallmark intellectual debates as Du Bois, Booker T. Washington and Marcus Garvey, Martin Luther King

Jr. and Malcolm X, and, even more recently, Louis Farrakhan, Jesse Jackson Sr., and Barack Obama. Obama, although largely characterized as the quintessential Black leader for his ascension to the US presidency, has been critiqued for his seemingly playing respectability politics in his notions toward Black masculinity. More telling, however, is how many key figures that offered polarizing and complex views of Black masculinity have been marginalized from the larger discussion of Black masculine leadership, including names such as Huey P. Newton, Fred Hampton, Bayard Rustin, and James Baldwin. Newton and Hampton, both leaders within the Black Panther Party, were noted for their keen intellect, charisma, and socialist political framing. Both considered radicals in the historical view, along with Malcolm X, they were seen as militant and untenable to the larger Black community and consequently US mainstream consumption. Rustin, as both gay and socialist, known as the mastermind behind such seminal events as the 1963 March on Washington, was kept in the margins by his contemporaries and, until recently, left out of the larger conversation concerning Black leadership (Morgan, 2020). Baldwin, on the other hand, although accepted as an award-winning author, was marginalized among civil rights discourse as well because of his effeminate presence. These examples are very telling in exploring Black masculinity.

For Newton and Hampton, Black masculinity that seeks to upend power boldly, unapologetically Black, and outspoken concerning class struggles, particularly the Black elite, were deemed a threat to both the white and Black establishment and ultimately left alone to deal with the onslaught of US terror. For Rustin and Baldwin, their intellectual and social movement prowess was marginalized due to their contradicting of the traditional notions of Black masculinity—cisgender, patriarchal, and dominant—and thus not good examples of Black men in leadership. Taking an intersectionalist approach, it is clear to see that all four men were complex figures who went beyond traditional tropes of masculinity. Both Newton and Hampton spoke out against all oppression and were inclusive of the gay and lesbian communities and formed multiracial alliances across social strata. Rustin and Baldwin were both courageous, strong, and charismatic, and although placed in the margins in the struggle, they were very much close compatriots of those men and women who held more traditional roles of masculinity and femininity, including King and Malcolm X.

The emergence of the #BlackLivesMatter movement has shed light on the marginalization of divergent identities throughout movement history, being both unapologetically Black and as well, visibly inclusive of the LGBTQ community, stating that *all* Black lives matter. Initiated because of the deaths of Black males Trayvon Martin, Michael Brown, Eric Gardner, and many others, gay, queer, and trans men have been at the forefront in different cities across the United States in bringing attention to police killings and the lack of equity in US society. Clear in their fight to stop the killing of Black men and boys by police, they also have been clear how they position their intersectional identities. This embrace of all of who they are, as well as all of who Black people are, allows for a framing for social workers to move beyond essentialist notions of the Black masculine toward a more inclusive paradigm that can affirm the many identities that Black men and boys hold.

Defining the Remix: Exploring Complex Identities Among Black Men and Boys

A "remix" is a term generally used in media that refers to taking an existing or original recording and providing or altering it via adding, taking away, or changing it in some way. Remixing can be applied to art, photographs, or video but is more popular within music. In this chapter, we consider how Black masculinity has been viewed in sociocultural and sociopolitical contexts, as well as within social science research and practice. The chapter then illustrates how social movements have attempted to value Black life, and thus Black masculinity, and how social science research and practice have struggled to illustrate this complexity. The authors hope to add to the social work canon of viewing Black masculinity as "masculinities," offering that a larger, more nuanced view of Black men and boys can understand both shared and divergent views of Black masculinity and thus more effectively intervene, advocate, and support Black men and boys in social work settings.

The three case studies offered in this chapter can provide insight into this "remix," or how Black men and boys and intersectionality can work at the program level to enhance positive outcomes for individuals, families, and communities.

Case Studies

Connections

After leading a rites of passage (ROP) program for over ten years, I have recently begun to reflect on the identities that made up the various cohorts of adolescent Black males and females. The program was called Connections and anchored itself in an African cultural social ethos that promoted a sense of meaning and purpose. Warfield-Coppock (1992) describes the rites as a celebration or ceremony, and the passage refers to transition from stage to another; adolescence would be in the puberty stage. Puberty rites would indicate a society's acknowledgment that a child has reached the age of responsibility, fertility, and community productivity (Weisfeld, 1997). Connections used cultural awareness as a tool for self-awareness, and through that journey they would become more open to self-exploration. Connections was based in West Englewood, on Chicago's Southwest side which has been considered to be one of the most violent communities in the nation at one time. Many of the young men in the program had been either in a gang or gang affiliated. Ninety percent of the young men did not have the presence of a father in the household and were solely raised by their mother or in some cases grandmother.

Many of the young men were initially drawn to the Connections program because it seemed to have all the elements of a secret society. There was the element of familiarity as Connection members would greet each other in their Akan names in the hallway. Some would dress in an assortment of African garb and would at times speak in what seemed like another language. Connection members would blurt out phases like wo ho to sen, which means "how are you" in Twi to other members who would respond by saying Meda wo asa, meaning "I'm fine." The language was basic phrases from the Akan culture, and understanding the greetings was a staple of the ROP program. They were also intrigued by the element of respect as the elder man who helped to facilitate the program was called Baba which is a term of endearment and means father. They were also intrigued by the ritualistic aspect of the program. The rituals seemed like to them an initiatory process similar to what gang members would have to go through in order to join.

One student named Dante (pseudonym) was especially curious about the program and sat in the healing circles with the other members and would ask pointed questions after each session. *Why do you let them see you cry? Why do you trust these people like that, you don't know them. Why do you act differently in the circle?* Eventually Dante joined Connections and quickly became one the leaders. Dante found comfort with the Connection members accepting him and not judging him. Dante was struggling with his sexual identity and presented as a cisgender male. In the masculinity formation, Dante would be categorized as subordinate who was in contention with the hegemonic or dominant male role. Gause (2008) calls this the "masking strategy" where in his desire to exhibit masculinity he has to deny or suppress his feelings. Gause (2008) goes on to say, "The only way for black males to transcend the hegemonic construction of their masculinity and overcome these masking strategies is to seek new constructions by using the historical narratives of their brothers and sisters to construct new narratives of liberation. This requires a critical understanding of the spiritual self" (p. 159). Gause believes that African Americans must engage in a critical spirituality process, one that engages in "critical self-reflection, deconstructive interpretation, performative creativity, and transformative action" (Dantley, 2007, p. 160). The Afro cultural-focused rites of passage provides that spiritual space. Lance Williams (2010) points out that "spirituality is central in African-centered ontology, cosmology, and axiology; in its ideology, ethos, and worldview; and in adherents' behavior, values, and attitudes. Therefore where there is African culture in any form, there is spirituality" (p. 279).

Williams (2010) concludes that cultivating spirituality among the participants was a critical part of the program. This was done through rituals such as the pouring of libation which allows for one's ancestors to be invited in and honored. Connection participants perceived themselves to be protected by their ancestors, which allowed them to steer clear of risky behavior. Smudging was also utilized, which symbolized the process of a spiritual cleansing of a sacred ritual space (ibid., 280). These rituals were important as they provided the communal space and energy that allowed for the participants to expand their awareness and undergo transformation. The Connections program provided a variety of approaches to help the males in the program to cope with stress, frustration, and anger. One such process was referred to as clearing, which was a facilitated process to move "inward" to confront past emotionally traumatic experiences. Dante described the Stick-Action Ritual:

If I had a conflict with another group member, I would probably go to Z or one of the elders, which is something people always do….So, they'll (the elders) get the stick and put it in the center of the room. Everyone would gather in a circle around, you know, just as support. I would be on one side of the stick and the other person …(would be on the other side). Yeah, I would call the person that I was in a conflict with ….I would say to the person, "You have to come to the stick" I would ask the person "Can you do this?"

And the person would say, "Yeah, I'll do it," "Yeah it's cool."….So then I tell them what happened, you know….I would just basically clear my stuff off with the person in the presence of the group and the elders. But the stick is not goin' directly at the person, all this negative feelings is goin' in the ground. The whole piece I'm doing….Basically the person is just a mirror for me. It's not really the person, it's about me…. (Williams, 2010)

The clearing process emboldened Dante and gave him a voice. Jackson and Elmore (2017) note that this type of recognition helps to define the role of masculinity. Jackson and Elmore (ibid) argue that "the process of one's behavior being recognized allows for the validation of the individual to be seen as masculine."

A stage of the ROP allows for the participant to receive their Akan name. By using a perpetual calendar, Connection members were able to find the day of the week that aligns with their Akan birth name. Dante's is Kwabena, a Tuesday's child whose attributes are as follows:

- "Manly," full of fire and determination. A risk taker and bold, who is a source of inspiration for others
- Risk, letting go of familiar protective identity to stay on purpose.

The naming ceremony provided confirmation on how Dante and others in the group saw Dante in his masculine identity. Dante found a measure of solace in the Connections program, which afforded him the opportunity to have a sense of agency and to demonstrate his natural leadership skills. Dante has been able to negotiate his identity and masculinity by seeing through a nurturing African cultural lens. Dante had begun to address what psychologist Shanette M. Harris regards as the "Compensation for feelings of insecurity in a Eurocentric world that's led the African-American male particularly the youth to redefine what it means to be a man in the present world" (Harris, 1995).

Truth N' Trauma

The Truth n' Trauma Program (TNT) was developed to address the impact of exposure to violence on African American youth via utilizing a trauma-informed, restorative, and culturally affirming intervention to promote healing and social action (Harden et al., 2015). All young people involved were offered a trauma-informed workshop created by Dr. Kimberly Mann, then designer of trauma-informed training for the Illinois Department of Children and Family Services. The trauma training included six modules of intensive trauma training, including the impact of violence exposure on individuals, families, and communities and strategies for healing. Youth involved also went through critical consciousness and restorative practices training, along with cultural awareness education. Youth were then engaged in four tracks: trauma workshop creation and leadership, participatory action research, theater, and documentary filmmaking.

Products were created for their peers and others who were interested in learning more about both the impact of violence and pathways toward healing. The program was intentional concerning recruitment of an equal number of young men and women, and they differed in respect to their school and extracurricular involvement and overall backgrounds. All were African American and from the south side of Chicago, Illinois, and although several went on to college, including such places as Harvard and West Point, some were street organization affiliated and had multiple arrests. The young people were encouraged to choose any of the four tracks that they felt most interested. The majority of the young men chose the video documentary and the trauma workshop creation groups. In the theatre group, there were nine young women and four young men. One product for creation was a play entitled "The Only Way Out Is Through." The following discusses the impact of the track on the young people and one young man in particular.

"Dude disappeared fuh ah lil while doe"

The participants involved in the theater component grew close through the dramaturgical process, including spending time with each other prior to rehearsal to "check in" in a restorative circle fashion. They also took time to journal, of which some of their writings were turned into aspects of the performance they created. The play created came from a mixture of their discussions related to the exposure of violence young African Americans experience, including the historical and political aspects of living while Black in America. One young woman, in a part of the performance, recited a poem she created, while her peers performed tableaux accenting her words.

The ensemble performed "The Only Way Out Is Through" on multiple occasions, including at Activist/Professor Bill Ayers's house as part of the Chicago Home Theater Festival; at the Jane Addams Hull House as the evening's headliners in the Building Peace and Justice Series; and at the Illinois Childhood Trauma Coalition's Symposium on Child Trauma in the Public Sector, the first performance ever featured at this conference. By traditional standards of social service intervention, including program evaluation and public opinion, the program and the play was a success (Harden, 2017). However, as with most programs like this, mistakes, failures, and lessons learned were an important part of the process. Youth who start in a program, and do not always remain or even if they stay involved, can fall back into patterns that undermine their individual and collective process. In addition, violence and issues of racial equity continue to be ongoing problems in many cities, more a failure not of programming, but the daunting systemic racism that these programs are initiated to supposedly address. Most revealing of this was the process of witnessing the success of "The Way Through" and the challenges associated with keeping young men engaged in social programs.

One of the young women participants, in writing a journal entry, shared:

> Theatre. Take time to understand how we made it this far. Ok ladies. Viewpointing. Female issues. Attitude. Damn why did I choose this group? What the hell. No shoes well ok I guess I can do that. No socks. Aw hell nhaw. My toes ain't done 'n my feet ashy. Get use to the process but not the people. Damn did she just roll her eyes at me? 9 girls 4 boys. Shidd was his reason for not coming. Viewpointing everybody. Now let's begin gestures. 9 girls 3 boys. Dude disappeared fuh ah lil while doe. Viewpoints everybody. Fast is fast. Slow is slow. You're either up in the sky or down on the floor. Topography you know. Move around. Touch it don't be scared. 9 girls 2 boys. Wait was he even here to begin with? Shidd guess it's time for the real thing. Practice makes perfect. We may need to meet on Monday and stay longer on Saturdays. 9 girls1 boy. Is where we are today. Ensemble is what you call it. Attitudes bonded together. Writing, crying, sharing.... Thanks. Cus if it wasn't for y'all my mask would still be on. (Martinson, 2015, pp. 156–157)

Her writing, although speaking about her own internal struggle, reveals her mixed feelings about being active in the program but also speaks to her struggle associated with Black male presence. She notes the decline in male participation as a countdown from four boys, to two, and then finally to one, questioning in the end, "Wait was even here to begin?" The statement "Dude disappeared fuh ah lil while doe" also reveals a critical component often left out of youth and intervention literature: why some young people are consistent and others seemingly inconsistent. Although there can be a number of reasons for this inconsistency, telling is what one of the program leaders had to say. In an article reflecting on this, the Theatre Dramaturg supervising the play, Karen Jean Martinson (2015), writes:

> Our final male was the most upsetting. His personal life was difficult: he was temporarily homeless, had little family support, and had to cross multiple gang lines to get to campus— and, in the parlance of the South Side, he had been 'jumped on' as a result. When present, he was committed and inventive and contributed greatly to the devising process. Yet, the unpredictability of his life made his attendance erratic. (p. 156)

Although the program was decidedly trauma-informed and culturally relevant, it could not compete with the day-to-day obstacles that this young man encountered. In his "ghosting," an important part of the play developed, connecting his presence/ absence with the lives of Emmett Till, Trayvon Martin, and other Black boys who could not be protected. Unlike Trayvon and Teal, he was not murdered; however, he faced the greater threats of violence that young Black men his age face. As a part of one young man's monologue for the play, this determination yet loss is portrayed, as the monologue consisted of both the young man who was no longer a part of the ensemble, below in gray, and the young man who remained:

> NO. Move around because your faker than artificial. I'm authentic and official, and for the bullshit, I keep tissue. I try, he try, we try ... But still my brothers are claimed. (Martinson & Jackson, 2015, p. 276)

This young man was not the "star" of the ensemble, as his performative absence was neither seen nor felt by the audience. In addition, he was not highlighted at the beginning of the program by his popularity or his street presence: he was just another Black boy. However, it was clear that his presence was felt by his peers, and the impact of his loss from the program was felt by all. This illustrates a clear dilemma in programming for Black males: young Black men who are the most "at-risk" are often focused upon, and many fall through the cracks due to a lack of attention. Other young men, those who are consistent, have the markings of success, including academic, athletic, or social performance, and are highlighted and fast tracked toward success, often supported by multiple allies in the process. The remaining male went on to reflect later:

> We lost so many people, so many males within our group, we finally get one who writes something, and he's gone! So it was just like, can I just let him go like that? Like … that's all my point. Everybody's like, am I my sister's keeper, or, am I my brother's keeper? Do I just let his stuff go like that? Or do I really try to get it into myself and really put him on the stage? You don't have to see him to see … him. You don't have to see Trayvon to see Trayvon. (A. Al-Hassan, personal communication, February 20, 2014, in Martinson & Jackson, 2015, p. 276)

Metropolitan Peace Academy

The Metropolitan Peace Academy (MPA) is a part of the Communities Partnership for Peace Initiative (CP4P) at Metropolitan Family Services in Chicago. It was designed to promote professionalism for street outreach workers via trauma-informed, restorative, and hyper-local curriculum. The majority of MPA participants were former street organization leaders, many of whom had served significant time in correctional facilities. Most were employed at agencies that address community violence, who had also been connected to other efforts to interrupt the cycle of violence, including Cure Violence (formerly Ceasefire), the Institute for Nonviolence, and other well-known violence intervention organizations. The curriculum was developed by the author and leaned heavily on lessons learned in the application of the previous case studies, including the importance of building community, cultural affirmation, and leadership development.

One of the participants, called here "Roscoe," came to MPA as a part of its first cohort. Previously employed with Cure Violence, he was terminated after recidivating based on an acknowledged mistake: participating in a crime that would also violate his parole. After serving a few years, he returned to work at a violence intervention agency as an outreach worker but was uncertain of his future and contemplated returning to crime. Roscoe was a respected leader in his street organization, where he was initiated into while in middle school, slowly moving up to "shot caller" status. Although working for an agency, he presented as "rough-around-the-edges," and few organizational supervisors tapped him for leadership potential within their agencies. Sensing this, Roscoe was mostly ambivalent concerning his commitment level, recognizing that there was little future in the hierarchy of the organization as well as the larger world of violence interruption and street outreach. Although a "credible messenger," someone seen as having the ability to men, women, and children still involved in violent activities but with street credibility to be trusted enough to share positive messages to those still involved. Roscoe was a valuable frontline worker but not valuable enough to be mentored toward leading efforts for larger community change. This dynamic is seen throughout the profession.

When talking with Roscoe one day, a new story related to a political figure became a point of discussion. Roscoe thoroughly dissected the issue, and when asked how he knew so much, he shared that he read five newspapers daily: *The Tribune*, the *Sun-Times*, The *Wall Street Journal*, the *New York Times*, and *Crain's*. Soon, staff at the MPA began calling Roscoe "The Professor," a nickname referencing his deep analysis of complex policy, organizational, and social issues. Roscoe later went on to not only complete the MPA but also became a leader in Chicago addressing gun violence.

Implications for Practice

Social workers have the unique opportunity of engaging participants based on the context of their circumstances, as Bryan Stevenson, founder of the Equal Justice Project and author of *Just Mercy: A story of justice and redemption* stated, "Each of us is more than the worst thing we've ever done" (Stevenson, 2015, p. 17). Many Black men and boys come into programming after being referred for behaviors that are outside of the social norm. In remixing a traditional heteronormative and respectability politics and essentialist view of Black masculinity, we contend that the Black male experience has always been complex, nuanced, and inclusive of intersectional identities of Black men and boys. A remixed lens calls for the integration of the sociopolitical, historical, cultural, and intersecting identities reflective of the complex identities of Black men and boys. The case studies illustrate how seeing these young men in a "both/and" approach, recognizing the context surrounding their Blackness and also the individual expressions of identity that can be marginalized in the settings for needs-based programming. Programs that seek to engage Black men and boys often homogenize the intersectional aspects in order to fit into a one-size-fits-all programming frame. By accepting at program onset that all Black men and boys are unique and comprising of a range of the Black male experience, social workers can move beyond traditional approaches to cultural competence and challenge funder and policy maker suggestions. For example, when designing the peace academy, program administrators pressured curriculum designers to dumb-down the curriculum, stating that the literacy levels of many of the men, often high school drop outs who spent several years incarcerated, could not keep up with rigorous curriculum. Although some of this was true for some of the participants, it did not account that some of the participants were not only college graduates but also possessors of graduate degrees and, in Roscoe's case, voracious consumers of media and literal text.

In including the cultural, historical, and sociopolitical, programming can also be "honest" in nature, not highlighting a certain type of Blackness but an inclusive

Black masculinity that can highlight not only a Dr. King or Malcolm X as a role model but also a James Baldwin, Larry Hoover, and Huey P. Newton.

Summary

All three case studies, illustrating programs designed at different times for Black men and adolescents, demonstrate the complex interactions that take place for providers and their participants. All, interdisciplinary in nature, were led by social workers trained in traditional social work practices from major social work institutions. However, the providers were also steeped in knowledge related to African-centered practice, including African Rites of Passage processes, restorative justice, trauma-informed care, and Black sociopolitical education, not taught in these programs at the time. Their additional training allowed them to be flexible, nuanced, and integrative in approaches that best fit both the larger sociopolitical context and the individuals present in their respective programs. Adhering to only an evidence-based framework would not have allowed for the innovation needed to support these young people in a true social work framing: "Meeting the client where they are at." Going beyond this as well, leaders also included the "at" to involve the complex structural issues reflected by racism, patriarchy, heteronormativity, and classism in particular. However, this did not necessarily mean all efforts were 100% successful for all of the youth. Included within the larger tale successes are also mistakes, heartbreaking moments, and lessons learned. Social work programs should be inclusive of these aspects of their programming as well; in situating narratives as either successful or failed, do not allow for the level of complexity, innovation, and sustainability needed to address at times overwhelming social problems. In addition, programs that are led by African Americans are not always given the bandwidth to "fail," and providers force programs into highlighting only success stories, shaped based on a certain type of young person, usually an individual who meets the criteria of respectability. All three case studies illustrate young men who were not "typical" but reflect their own variation of Black masculinity and intersecting identities that contextualize who they are. Martinson's words, although discussing theater, gives us some insight here: "Crafting a piece grounded in a dramaturgy of failure—a dramaturgy that actively disrupts notions of suffering and victimhood—helps to navigate hope, preventing it from becoming too sweet and easy" (2015, p. 150). Seeing them only through one lens as "endangered" would not allow for insights to emerge as not only clients in need of care but future leaders toward the development of other Black males. Their stories illustrate how talent is often unseen by both institutional bias and by choice, and methods to engage in traditional ways fail to engage them in effective programming. We do not "see" the Trayvon Martins, Lacquan McDonalds, Ahmaud Arberys, or George Floyds until they're gone, but if we perhaps look harder, they are around us all the time.

Discussion Questions

1. What assumptions do you carry about Black men and boys that come from your personal and professional experiences?
2. What common characteristics do you believe exist among Black men and boys?

3. What are the divergent "types" of Black men and boys you encounter? In what ways did you consider this has helped or harmed you in working with Black men and boys?
4. How might your programming be different if you take an intersectional approach to working with Black men and boys? What ways might you have to alter your current programming or remix methods and processes that you currently employ?
5. What types of training do you believe you and/or your staff need to effectively include an intersectional approach?
6. Who are some of the historical and professional images of Black men and boys that you can include in your presentation of Black men (for example, Black gay scientists, Black gang members who are book nerds, or Black male athletes who are into Anime)?

Glossary of Terms and Concepts

Intersectionality: the study of how overlapping social identities intersect and their related systems of oppressive institutions. Intersectionality theory proposes that the trait of a person is inextricably linked with all the other traits or elements to entirely recognize a person's identity and shared and lived experiences with others of comparable social identities.

Masculinity: a social descriptor that travels, with meaning varying by region, clan, family, and country.

Remix: taking an existing or original and altering it via adding, taking away, or changing it in some way. Remixing can be applied to art, photographs, or video but is more popular within music and in this case of viewing Black masculinity as "masculinities" Black men, racialized and historical trauma, and masculinity.

References

Bowleg, L., del Río-González, A. M., Holt, S. L., Pérez, C., Massie, J. S., Mandel, J. E., & Boone, C. A. (2017). Intersectional epistemologies of ignorance: How behavioral and social science research shapes what we know, think we know, and don't know about U.S. black men's sexualities. *The Journal of Sex Research, 54*(4–5), 577–603. https://doi.org/10.1080/0022449 9.2017.1295300

Connell, R. (1995). *Masculinities.* University of California Press.

Crenshaw, K. (1989). Demarginalizing the intersection of race and sex: A Black feminist critique of antidiscrimination doctrine, feminist theory and antiracist politics, in *University of Chicago Legal Forum, 8*(1), 139–167.

Dantley, M. (2007). Re-radicalizing the consciousness in educational leadership: The critically spiritual imperative toward keeping the promise. *Counterpoints, 305*, 159–176. Retrieved May 10, 2021, from http://www.jstor.org/stable/45136059

Dean, J. J. (2013). Heterosexual masculinities, anti-homophobias, and shifts in hegemonic masculinity: The identity practices of black and white heterosexual men. *Sociological Quarterly, 54*(4), 534–560.

DuBois, W. E. B. [1903] (1999). *The souls of black folk.* Bantam Books.

Engle, J. (2018). *500 years of black resistance.* Downloaded from website https://decolonialatlas. wordpress.com/2018/02/18/500-years-of-black-resistance/. May 1, 2021.

Fine, M. (1990). Making controversy: Who's "at risk"? *Journal of Cultural Studies, 1*(1), 55–68.

Gause, C. (2008). Chapter 1: Integration matters. *Counterpoints, 337*, 15–36. Retrieved May 10, 2021, from http://www.jstor.org/stable/42979204

Graves Holmes, G. (1994). Recontextualizing black resistance: A review essay. *Eighteenth-Century Studies, 28*(1), 141–144.

Griffith, D. M., Gunter, K., & Watkins, D. C. (2012). Measuring masculinity in research on men of color: Findings and future directions. *American Journal of Public Health, 102*(S2), 187–196.

Harden, T. (2017). We still cool? Revisiting black masculinity, and urban violence in Brooks' "we real cool". In Q. Lasana (Ed.), *The whiskey of our discontent*. Haymarket Press.

Harden, T., Kenemore, T., Mann, K., Edwards, M., List, C., & Martinson, K. J. (2015). The truth n' trauma project: Addressing community violence through a youth-led, trauma-informed, restorative framework. *Child and Adolescent Social Work Journal, 32*, 65–79.

Harris, S. M. (1995). Psychosocial development and black male masculinity: Implications for counseling economically disadvantaged African American male adolescents. *Counseling and Development, 73*(3), 279–287.

Jackson, R. L., II, & Elmore, B. (2017). Black masculinity. In Y. Y. Kim (Ed.), *The international encyclopedia of intercultural communication*. Wiley Blackwell.

Majors, R., & Billson, J. M. (1992). *Cool pose: The dilemmas of black manhood in America*. Lexington.

Martinson, K. J. (2015). "The way through": Social action and the critical embrace of failure. *Theatre Topics, 25*(2), 149–160.

Martinson, K. J., & Jackson, G. (2015). Ain't that a shame? Trayvon's trauma revealed through the theatre of TNT. *Cultural Studies ↔ Critical Methodologies, 15*(4), 271–277.

Morgan, T. (2020). Why MLK's right-hand man was nearly written out of history. *HISTORY*. Retrieved April 19, 2021 https://www.history.com/news/bayard-rustin-march-on-washington-openly-gay-mlk

Stevenson, B. (2015). *Just mercy: A story of justice and redemption*. Spiegel & Grau.

Swadener, B. B. (1995). Children and families "at promise": Deconstructing the discourse of "at-risk". In B. B. Swadener & S. Lubek (Eds.), *Children and families "at promise"*. SUNY Press.

Unnever, J. D., & Chouhy, C. (2020). Race, racism, and the cool pose: Exploring white and black male masculinity. *Social Problems, 0*, 1–23. https://doi.org/10.1093/socpro/spaa010

Warfield-Coppock, N. (1992). The rites of passage movement: A resurgence of African-centered practices for socializing African American youth. *Journal of Negro Education, 61*(4), 471–482.

Weisfeld, G. (1997). Puberty rites as clues to the nature of human adolescence. *Cross-Cultural Research, 31*(1), 27–54.

Williams, L. (2010). Cultural interventions for reducing violence among young African American males. In W. E. Johnson (Ed.), *Social work with African American males: Health, mental health, and social policy*. Oxford University Press.

Young, A. A. (2017). The character assassination of black males: Some consequences for research in public health. In K. Bogard, V. M. Murry, & C. Alexander (Eds.), *Perspectives on health equity and social determinants of health* (pp. 110–115). National Academy of Medicine.

Troy Harden,   PhD, LCSW, has over 25 years' experience working in higher education and community settings. His ongoing research interests are in racial equity, community violence, social trauma, and interventions within community and organizational settings. He recently developed and led Northeastern Illinois University's Master of Social Work program in Chicago, and is now Director of the Race and Ethnic Studies Institute (RESI) and faculty in the Department of Sociology at Texas A & M University in College Station. He has worked closely with Communities Partnering for Peace (CP4P), an effort to develop violence interventions for African American and Latino street outreach workers addressing violence in Chicago. As well, he is the lead researcher with the Department of Justice, Bureau of Justice Assistance's Community-based Crime Reduction Grant in Englewood, partnering with the Englewood Public Safety Task Force. He has served as a leadership consultant with multiple institutions on issues of race, gender and poverty, including the City of Chicago's Department of Family Support Services; the Latino Policy Forum; Chicago Public Schools; Fathers, Families, and Healthy Communities; the Pan African Association; the Illinois African American Coalition for Prevention; Burrell Communications and Cook County's Project Brotherhood, a Black men's health clinic. He is also Board President of the Chicago Torture Justice Center, which provides mental health and community services for survivors of police torture by Chicago Police Commander Jon Burge and others impacted by state-sponsored violence. He received an outstanding educator award from Congressman Danny K. Davis in 2017, is a graduate of Loyola University Chicago's Master of Social Work program, and received his doctorate from DePaul University's School of Education.

John Zeigler Jr., MSW, is the Director of the Egan Office of Urban Education and Community Partnerships (UECP) at DePaul University in Chicago, Illinois. He provides guidance on UECP's role in advancing an activist scholarship with DePaul faculty and students on engagement with public agencies, community-based organizations and schools. John recognized that the most effective solutions to community issues should be community-driven. For over 25 years, John has been a researcher, community organizer, and counselor. He's the founder of the African-centered Rites of Passage program called Connextions, which was designed to develop adolescents into conscious community builders. For over 12 years, these students from Chicago's South Side traveled to West Africa, where they went through a rites-of-passage process.

John is senior advisor for the Goldin Institute's Chicago Peace Fellows, where he assists and guides global and local grassroots organizations in building collaborative peacebuilding projects. He has been a critical voice in the construction of organizations such as Southwest Youth Services Collaborative; Chicago Survivors; Young Chicago Authors; Fathers, Families and Healthy Communities; and the Rites of Passage program for Chicago CRED (Create Real Economic Destiny).

John received his Master of Social Work from the University of Illinois in Chicago and is adjunct faculty at DePaul University and the Asset-Based Community Development Institute (ABCDI). He is currently finishing his doctorate in education where his research interest is authentic participation of black community-based organizations in the privatized environment of public schools.

Chapter 7
Building a Movement with Black Men: Culture Is the Key

Jerry Watson and Gregory Washington

> *Until the lion tells the story, the hunter will always be the hero.*
>
> *African Proverb*

The room was packed with families, friends, and community members. A haunting and eerie silence permeated the air. Many of the guests had never experienced anything of the sort. It was a rare event, and the crowd appeared mesmerized by the African drums playing a hypnotic, soft, and slow beat. The men (initiates) entered the room one by one, alone, and visibly shaken. Each man walked slowly across the room to meet with a small group of elders. To maintain privacy and secrecy, they spoke softly so that no one outside of their group could hear what they were saying. And after a brief pause of silence, a deep, loud, booming, and resounding voice from the group of elders proclaimed, "I introduce to you a man!" The crowd yelled in relief, clapped with approval, and screamed in the sweetness of African tones to mark the joy of the beginning of a journey into manhood. Once again, the room settled down and returned to a calm silence with the exception of the drums.

Now finally it was my turn "to go through the door." I didn't have a clue about the next challenge. Not knowing what was on the other side of the door, I felt fear, confusion, and fatigue from the two days of challenges, rituals, and compulsory activities. I walked slowly through the door following hand signals to join the small group of elders. What would happen now? I stood silently in anticipation of the unknown. I began to physically tremble and shake. After a brief private discussion and questioning, I was instructed to turn and face the crowd. Out of the silence, a deafening but clear voice roared, "I introduce to you a man!" When the congratulatory and sycophantic antics calmed, I heard a voice say, "He waited until he was 40 years old to become a man!" I was embarrassed and ashamed by the remark, but I

J. Watson (✉) · G. Washington
School of Social Work, University of Memphis, Memphis, TN, USA
e-mail: Jwtson28@memphis.edu; Gwshngt1@memphis.edu

knew it was the truth. My life would never be the same after coming through the door that evening. Little did I know that I would go through several more doors in the quest to become the person I was born to be.

The Need for Rites of Passages: "A Strengths-Based Approach to Working with Black Men"

Madhubuti (1991) explained that the pain is in their eyes. Young Black men in their late 20s or early 30s living in America, abandoned, aimlessly walking and hawking the streets with nothing behind their ears but anger, confusion, disappointment and pain. These men, running the streets, "lamping", occupying street corners, are beaten beyond recognition, with scars both visible and invisible. These men, Black men – sons of Africa, once strong and full of strength and hope that America lied about – are now knee-less, voice broken, homeless, forgotten, and terrorized into becoming beggars, thugs, drug addicts, alcoholics, thieves, or ultra-dependents on a system that considers them less than human and treats them with less respect than dead dogs (Madhubuti, 1991).

Understanding that the transatlantic slave trade, the Jim Crow era, and institutionalized oppression have fostered self-concepts of inferiority, cultural incompetence, and maladaptive behavior that influence African Americans (Serpell et al., 2009; Whaley & Noel, 2012; Washington et al., 2017), it became clear that a new approach was required. African-centered rites of passage interventions are in part inspired by beliefs that people of African descent continue to have the wisdom of elders and other African assets to overcome the influences of historical trauma along with developmental issues. Researchers have recommended that interventions for Black men should intentionally utilize the cultural assets of the African American community (Caldwell & White, 2001).

Social workers, ministers, responsible citizens, and parents are painfully aware of the recurrent and seemingly unsolvable problems and deplorable conditions they face daily. When the symbols, rituals, and cultural practices of a people's culture lose their legitimacy and power to compel thought and action, then disruption occurs within the cultural orientation and reflects itself as pathology in the people belonging to that culture (Nobles et al., 1987). What happens is that we create our own symbols, norms, values, rituals, colors, and activities and ascribe meaning to them. More often than not, these efforts are self-destructive and counter-productive to the health of the people, families, communities, and nation. Gangs, cliques, or street organizations provide the structure and processes simulating rites of passages for many young Black males. These groups serve as a surrogate support community for Black males by providing the essential elements for a negative rewarding existence. These groups or social networks are self-destructive in nature, yet provide rules or laws, meaning, direction, missions, symbols, significance, and a sense of belonging and connectedness while hiding the certain destructive end to themselves and others.

Similarly, for many Black men, mass incarceration has become a setting for socialization, for learning how to live, grow, and relate to others. Values and norms learned behind bars often accompany those who return to the community (Potts, 2013). The journey "in, out, and back in again" of prison resembles a revolving door for Black men. Potts posits that Black men find themselves not only locked up in jail but also locked in the cycle of return to the prison system. Removal from this cycle mandates more than a physical exit or the threat of more stringent sentences. Of course, opportunities for healthy resettlement in society, including safe and affordable housing, employment, education, training, psycho-social support, and often mental health services, are compulsory to interrupt recidivism. In addition, Potts is clear that possibly, and more importantly, these men must address the need to spiritually and psychologically break the grip of behaviors, beliefs, attitudes, and ways of thinking that support and drive them to remain in the cycle of incarceration.

Mensah (n.d.) reminds us that in African culture and in many other communities, societies undertake an assortment of rites or rituals to facilitate and ensure the successful movement and entry into new life situations. The rites clarify the new role, responsibilities, and duties and mark a successful transition and departure from a disturbing and often confusing life crisis. Somé (1993) suggests that ritual is required as a remedy for such a dysfunctional and debilitating state of affairs. Somé declares that one must first locate its hidden area, its symbolic dimension, work with it first, and then assist in the restoration of the physical (visible) reality. Visible wrongs have the roots in the world of the spirit. To deal only would their visible presence is like trimming the leaves of a weed when you mean to uproot it. Rituals are the mechanism that uproots these dysfunctions. Rituals offer a realm in which the invisible portion of the dysfunction is worked on in ways that impact the seen (Somé, 1993; Potts, 2013).

Rites of passages as a cultural strength help interpret existence, organize life, and incorporate the combination of racial and ethnic values and ideas learned, shared, and communicated from generation to generation (Gusfield, 2006; Laitin & Weingast, 2006; Song, 2009; Washington et al., 2017). While celebrating cultural strengths has influenced the growth of interest in African-centered rites of passage interventions, some persistent challenges also impel interest. Historical trauma, racial bias, and cultural suppression in African and African American history have influenced interest in culturally centered rites of passage programs (Harvey & Coleman, 1997; Harvey & Rauch, 1997; Washington et al., 2017).

A Strengths-Based Approach

The strengths-based approach builds on the strengths of clients. When we view individuals as having latent strengths, resources, and assets, including their culture, we will also see their positive potential and resilience when they are in adverse conditions (McCashen, 2005). Two principles are fundamental to the strengths-based approach when working with Black men: (1) The belief that Black men have strengths and (2) that identifying, sharing, and mobilizing their strengths is key to building and creating positive personal, professional, and community growth and change. Needless to say, it is the social worker's responsibility to work in collaboration with Black men to awaken them so they may identify for themselves the various strengths that lie within. The strengths-based approach facilitates healing, balance, and purpose and is a radical departure from the mindset that has traditionally viewed them as deviant and dangerous (Saleebey, 2002). Utilizing the strengths-based approach is an empowering and liberatory praxis.

Culture as a Strength

The enslavement of Blacks in the North American colonies left a lasting system of racial oppression in the United States (Feagin, 2006; Johnson & Carter, 2020). People of African descent (i.e., Black Americans) continued to be subjugated to unfair treatment and social and economic oppression (Feagin, 2006). In the United States, Blacks were originally thought to be culturally deficient, and therefore, any common practices among them were considered byproducts of treatment and interactions with Whites (Gutman, 1976). Similarly, Hill (1992) explained that Black men have been labeled as dangerous, obsolete, at risk, and endangered. It is instructive to understand that the portrait of Black men has been painted and externally determined by the circumstances of their existence in the United States and framed by historic racism. Despite these transgressions, Johnson and Carter (2020) hypothesized that health-promoting aspects of Black racial identity (e.g., racial centrality), racial socialization (e.g., cultural socialization), and racism-related coping (e.g., confrontation), as well as higher levels of communalism and spirituality, would indicate one latent factor, Black cultural strength. Black Americans have persisted through centuries of oppression in North America. To survive, they retained Africultural values and adopted group-specific practices. Black cultural values and practices can potentially, if utilized, improve the well-being of the population. Notably, the National Alliance on Mental Health (NAMI) identified the following strengths:

- Black culture brings to bear on the healing process related to mental health.
- Traditional practices in African American community.
- The Church is a strong source of cultural support.
- Our tolerance for "being different" is much more than mainstream audience.
- Resiliency and forgiveness – hopeful. It takes a strength/skill set to see the odds and still have the expectation that things will improve.
- Discipline and perseverance.
- Commitment and passion.
- The spiritual part of African Americans allows connection to core strengths and skill sets
- Self-directed (NAMI, n.d.).

Understanding the critical usefulness of an Afrocentric cultural strengths-based approach (Stepteau-Watson et al., 2014), we proposed using cultural strengths as the framework for working with young Black males in reentry. The Afrocentric perspective acknowledges and encourages the use of African culture as a strength to promote resiliency. Utilizing the perspective of culture as a strength helps social work practitioners solve pressing social problems that diminish human potential and preclude positive social change (CAU, 2021). Applying strengths-based principles with a focus on cultural strengths, the authors began to develop a movement, "Men Healing Men and Communities" (MHMCN).

Building a Movement Utilizing Cultural Strengths: Men Healing Men and Communities

Men Healing Men and Communities was formed in 2016 to utilize African-centered cultural strengths to plan, develop, implement, and evaluate health-promoting interventions and strategies to improve the quality of life for Black men and their communities. From the beginning, we were intentionally interested in building a movement. We identified and recruited Black men from diverse communities and professions, government agencies, and various stations of life to collaboratively develop and plan the movement. Early on in the organizing process, we conducted community and personal asset mapping exercises with participants. This set of activities provided opportunities for participants to identify their community and personal assets. The men identified a wide range of community assets, including churches, colleges and schools, businesses, churches, banks, restaurants, supermarkets, clothing stores, barbershops and beauty salons, police stations, parks and recreation centers, medical centers, and homes. The personal assets identified included their talents, special skills (mechanics, plumbing, sports), relationships (family and friends), hobbies, knowledge, cultural practices (spiritual, religious, and personal beliefs, values, rituals), educational background, and experiences. Following the suggestions of Snow (2004), we asked the questions, "What are some gifts you take for granted? If you asked someone, what some of your gifts are, what would the person say? What are some of your strengths and assets that you don't often use? What are some gifts in your family that were passed down to you through heredity? What are some of the gifts you have that most people have no idea of because they have not seen those gifts?"

To support our strengths-based approach, we developed the movement utilizing Karenga's (2008) African-centered cultural values and the seven principles of Kwanzaa:

Umoja – Means unity in Swahili. To work toward building and preserving unity at all levels of life, including our families, communities, and nation.

Kujichagulia – Self-determination. This value refers to defining for ourselves our destiny while telling our own stories.

Ujima – Translated as working together to improve ourselves and our communities. Ujima refers to assuming accountability and responsibility for the problems we face and the problems facing our sisters and brothers.

Ujamaa – Cooperative economics. Similar to Ujima, this principle refers to uplifting our community economically by practicing entrepreneurship, owning and operating businesses in our community, and profiting from our efforts together.

Nia – Means purpose. Not just any purpose but a targeted purpose to build our communities into healthy and safe spaces that support our healthy growth and development.

Kuumba – Means "creativity." It is important for us to be persistent and creative in our efforts to make our community beautiful and to improve the conditions in our communities through our work.

Imani – Faith. Realizing that our faith coupled with smart work has sustained us through a history of oppression, we must maintain strong faith, knowing that life for us is and will continue to improve (Karenga, 2008).

To facilitate the internalization of the principles, the seven principles were adopted as guiding principles of practice and discussed during each meeting. After a series of collaborative planning meetings, the group identified five clearly defined focus areas of interest utilizing culturally centered strengths-based strategies:

1. *To provide technical assistance and support to professionals, organizations, and communities (training, program evaluations, and consultation).* Participants expressed their dissatisfaction with previous training that appeared to be irrelevant to their needs and the needs of the families and communities in which they served. Participants identified the need for training using strengths-based, culturally sensitive, and asset-based approaches and materials.

2. *To conduct trauma-informed violence intervention and prevention training workshops.* The men were clearly aware that trauma and violence permeated their communities and their lives as Black men. They were interested in learning about trauma-informed approaches along with violence intervention and prevention efforts that actually work. They asked the question, "What can we do to stop the violence?" There was clearly an atmosphere of confusion, pain, and futility but hope was still alive. They voiced the belief that somehow, someway they could collectively work together to figure out what to do to prevent violence in their families and communities and effectively address the trauma already present among the people they serve.

3. *To provide ongoing peer support and mentoring for Black male practitioners.* A resounding majority of men admitted that they did not have mentors or mentor figures with whom they could confide in, ask for help, or follow as a guide to move forward in their personal lives as fathers, professionals, servants, and leaders. It was necessary to purposely build strong familial relationships through culturally appropriate group processes.

4. *To participate in community-based trauma, violence intervention, and prevention efforts and activities.* The men agreed that it was important for them to take active roles as participants and service recipients in ongoing community activities

addressing community-based trauma, violence intervention, and prevention. They decided that it was important for them to be present at violence response activities, including vigils, walks, rallies, and other events in response to community violence.

5. *To engage in policy and program development with partners.* The men expressed a desire to develop new policies, programs, and initiatives highlighting the positives of Black men. There was an interest in innovative and proven approaches to educate Black men on policies negatively impacting their life, including but not limited to prison reentry, criminal background record and expulsion and sealing, father's rights, and child support laws.

Through a consensus-building process, the participants decided on the mission and vision statements of MHMCN.

Mission
We are African American Men committed to healing and empowering our youth, families, and communities. We work together to build and empower healthy communities, prevent violence, and to reduce and ultimately eliminate trauma in our lives and among our youth, families, and communities.

Vision
We understand that violence and trauma are chronic conditions that can be successfully treated and prevented. "Our vision is healthy communities – thriving, safe, and secure".

- A place where "We are not afraid of our neighbors."
- A place where we feel safe and comfortable.
- A place where we participate in social, educational, and cultural activities together with our neighbors.
- A place where we live, play, work, and recreate.
- A place where we enjoy a sense of ownership.
- A place where we can experience a shared cultural identity.
- A place where we can maintain and honor our uniqueness and diversity.
- A place where "We know our neighbors".
- A place where we work together cooperatively to identify and solve our problems! (MHMCN Strategic Plan, 2015).

Men Healing Men and Communities Rites of Passages Experience (ROPE): A Strengths-Based Approach to Working with Black Men

With more than 50 years of combined rites of passages and initiatory experience in five states and two West African countries, the authors designed the MHMCN ROPE process. In consideration of the focus areas identified earlier by the men in

MHMCN during the collaborative planning sessions and the fundamental precepts of rites of passages, an integrated ROPE curriculum was developed. By now MHMCN membership consisted of a wide spectrum of Black men, including: community volunteers, ministers, concerned citizens, educators, social workers, an Afrocentric musician, historian, and griot, community organizers, social entrepreneurs, a governmental agency administrator, social work students, a not-for-profit executive, and a child and a juvenile criminal justice administrator. Fueled by the strengths of their African-centered cultural assets, the ROPE curriculum aimed to:

1. Support bonding and a sense of belonging to a positive and productive group, family, or community
2. Reinforce a strong connection to the Black community and its resources
3. Share knowledge about Black history to build cultural pride and awareness
4. Foster a sense of resilience and determination to equip participants to overcome the realities of racism and oppression
5. Increase technical knowledge related to providing quality services to individuals, families, groups, and communities
6. Create a positive support network to sustain mentorship relationships among members
7. Continue to share knowledge about and access to health-promoting personal and community resources

The group development and personal development areas of the ROPE were conducted using modified circle work principles and practices. Circle work is an ancient group process used for education, problem-solving, and community building attributed to first world nations that existed in the United States prior to conquest of Europeans. The ROPE group process operated using the following basic guidelines:

- The groups were conducted with participants arranged in a circle.
- The circle is considered a sacred space filled with safety, energy, and potential for group and individual growth.
- What is said in the circle remained in the circle (to maintain the sanctity of the space).
- Circle rules were established and agreed upon by consensus, including, but not limited to, respect for all circle members, honesty, and integrity, along with a willingness to speak your peace and to listen to others.
- The African drumming circle was utilized to ritually symbolize the opening of the circle followed by the libations ritual.
- The drumming circle also symbolized the closing of the circle and the completion of the ROPE.

Ultimately, the ROPE curriculum covered the following topical areas and subjects.

Group Development
A. The Nguzo Saba – Utilizing the seven principles of Kwanzaa as our personal and collective values.

B. Selecting group symbols and naming the group – Understanding that one's personal identity of the individual is born out their group membership. The ROPE participants selected the Adinkra symbols Akoben (the war horn), symbolizing readiness to move into action, and Sankofa (the bird looking backward), signifying the importance of understanding our history and culture, in order to move forward (Kuwornu-Adjaottor et al., 2016).

C. The group's rites of passages mission became "Responding to the call to action to go back and get our history and culture!"

D. Learning to participate and facilitate the libations ritual, thereby recognizing and honoring our African and African American ancestors, our family ancestors, and the spirits yet to be born.

E. The importance of dress for ritual and ceremonial events.

F. Africanizing traditions and holiday celebrations, including Kwanzaa and other culturally specific events that celebrate and present opportunities to include our heritage.

G. The meaning of colors and music, in particular African drumming, its history, and its usefulness in facilitating discussion and bringing people together by using African drumming circles.

H. A basic introduction to African world history with the objective of participants learning that our history does not begin in slavery.

Personal Development

I. Personal identity development examining "my multiple names," including nicknames, position titles, my given name, my first name, last name, and middle name. What does each of the names mean? The participant discovers an African or cosmic name using the perpetual calendar and the ancient names of the day of the week from the Akan nation in Ghana, West Africa. Using this information, the participants began to develop an awareness of themselves as their positive and affirmative life stories began to unfold.

J. Reflecting on participants' personal family history and genealogy, realizing that the family carries certain positive characteristics, behaviors, skills, knowledge, and personal assets from generation to generation.

K. The development of a group mission statement.

L. The development of a personal mission statement.

Professional Development

Didactic sessions were utilized to transfer knowledge about the following topic areas:

M. Adverse Childhood Experiences (ACEs) and a Pair of ACEs

N. The impact of trauma and trauma-informed care

O. Understanding the healthy development of Black males.

P. Group facilitation skills

Q. Key public policies negatively impacting Black men, including child custody rights and child support laws

R. Strategies and resources to reduce gun violence and domestic violence in Black communities

S. Maintaining peer support and mentoring relationships
T. Professional self-care
U. The importance of maintaining social support group activities, i.e., African drumming circles

Conclusion: Men Healing Men and Communities in Action

MHMCN sponsored Community African Drumming Circles to facilitate positive social support among members and community members. Located in community and university spaces, these activities provided opportunities for participants to learn about African culture while connecting with other Black men. These groups also served as information and resource sharing meetings including information on mental health services, food, clothing, housing, employment, education, training, and legal issues. Often guests with knowledge and access to goods and services in a particular area were brought in to educate the group on a particular area.

MHMCN partnered with the Center for the Advancement for Youth Development (CAYD) to create, plan, and offer a virtual Community Engagement Series. MHMCN recruited experts The series consisted of five 1.5-h workshop discussions covering the following topics: (1) African Americans in Agriculture – from Africa to America; (2) On Becoming Your Best Person; (3) Connecting the Dots: Participatory Asset-Mapping; (4) From the Ground Up, Fifty Years of Social Work; and (5) Healing Historical and Community Trauma.

Using partnerships and collaborations with other projects, MHMCN hosted and facilitated Barbershop Talks. In Black communities, barbershops are historically a sacred space for Black men. In barbershops, Black men feel comfortable and safe enough to sometimes share their private thoughts and feelings with their barber. Often the discussions are about race, politics, family, relationships, and a host of other sometimes controversial topics. Black men in barbershops also share information about employment opportunities, laws, medical issues, and resources available inside and outside the community. The Barbershop Talks events simulate actual neighborhood barbershops by enlisting barbers to provide free haircuts in community or university settings. The free haircuts proved to be effective recruitment incentives. While some participants were getting haircuts others were participating in an African drumming circle. The groups ceremoniously opened with the libations ritual. Topics ranged from prisoner reentry, fatherhood, finding and keeping employment, familial issues, living with a criminal background, stress management, and political issues.

Community Forum – MHMCN in partnership with CAYD sponsored a panel presentation and discussion on Gun Violence Intervention and Prevention. Three panelists, consisting of community violence prevention practitioners representing a Chicago not-for-profit organization and a Texas A&M sociology faculty person, presented their knowledge and experience in reducing violence in urban communities. The panel was followed by a community discussion hosted by MHMCN.

MHMCN organized and facilitated numerous Community Drumming Circles. These gatherings served as check-in experiences, energizers, information sharing opportunities, and social support experiences. Participants established new bonds with positive and supportive Black men and strengthened already existing relationships.

Movie Viewing and Discussion – MHMCN sponsored the viewing of the movie *The Work*, followed by the issues highlighted in the film. The group discussed the emotional vulnerability of incarcerated Black men, their willingness to confront one another, and their sincere desire to help each other.

"Finding the Silver Lining in a Cloud": MHMCN's COVID-19 Response
Utilizing the kuumba value of creativity, MHMCN developed a database of community citizens, families, organizations, service providers, volunteers, and federal, state, county, and city governmental employees to identify longstanding and pop-up resources for individuals and families in need. MHMCN partnered with CAYD and used an interactive webpage on the University of Memphis's website, emails, text messages, telephone calls, and Facebook post to identify and connect community residents to a wide range of resources. MHMCN connected individuals and organizations to COVID-19 testing and vaccinations, mental health services, rent assistance, food and clothing giveaways, and computer training. Finally, MHMCN's development of a virtual presence on social media by joining Facebook and creating a webpage/link on the University of Memphis-CAYD site allows us to stay in touch with participants and to connect with community residents in need of support or assistance. These platforms enabled us to tell our story and to connect with a larger audience.

Summary
Developing and implementing programs and services targeting Black men offers unique opportunities for creating and utilizing their culturally centered assets. Using the griot's voice, this chapter presents the experiences of Black male elders employing strengths-based approaches while working with Black men. African rituals, values, and rites of passages experiences provide a framework for planning and implementing a range of programmatic strategies impacting Black men. The chapter concludes with a brief description of the organization's kuumba or creative response to the COVID-19 pandemic.

Discussion Questions
Exercise: "From Ideas to Action"

Social workers have a responsibility to understand the client, despite differences in beliefs, values, or choices, and to empower them to make the best decisions for themselves (Wahler, 2012). You are working in a community setting as a social worker. Your duties include designing, facilitating, and overseeing social and recreational activities for young Black men during the summer. The Director notices that lately there has been an increase in the number of young fathers enrolled in the programs. You have been selected to develop and start a new project targeting young Black fathers.

1. Using culture as a strength and rites of passage as a group approach, identify the programmatic elements that you would include in a parenting (fatherhood) program targeting Black fathers between the ages of 16 and 22 years.
2. Develop and describe three types of community-based organizations you would recruit and partner with to make your fatherhood program a success.
3. Explain three ways that you can utilize rites of passages programming to support the young fathers in the community you are working in.
4. Identify three values listed in the chapter that might be useful for your program participants.
5. How might program participants utilize the values that you have identified?
6. Identify two values listed in the chapter that you think the participants would most likely select for themselves as young fathers.
7. Why would they select the values that you listed in Question #6?
8. What program activities would you plan for a program serving African American males returning from prison who could no longer meet face-to-face because of the pandemic? Explain your answer in detail.

Glossary of Terms and Concepts

Rites of passages: A system of practices, activities, and ceremonies that facilitate, mark, and aid the development and movement of a person from one stage of life to another stage of life, such as pregnancy, birth, adolescence, adulthood, old age, death, marriage, educational and professional progress.

Nguza saba: Seven principles or values of Kwanzaa that provide guidance and direction to African American growth and development; considered a cultural asset.

Griot: Historian or storyteller.

Cultural asset or strength: A positive and health-promoting value, practice, activity, service, and programming that honors and utilizes the culture of participants in a way that promotes the growth, development, and healing of the participants.

Libations: An important African ritual that recognizes ancestors, the cycle of life, the unity of community, African and African American history and connectedness, and the importance of African culture while engaging all group members/participants in collective participation.

References

Akoma Unity Center. (2021). Retrieved from https://akomaunitycenter.org/what-are-rites-of-passage-and-why-are-they-so-important/

Caldwell, L. D., & White, J. L. (2001). African-centered therapeutic and counseling interventions for African-American males. In G. R. Brooks & G. E. Good (Eds.), *The new handbook of psychotherapy and counseling with men: A comprehensive guide to settings, problems, and treatment approaches* (pp. 737–753). Jossey-Bass.

CAU. (2021). Clark Atlanta University, Whitney, M. Young School of Social Work. Retrieved from https://www.cau.edu/school-of-social-work/The-Afrocentric-Perspective.html

Feagin, J. R. (2006). *Systemic racism*. Routledge.

Gusfield, J. (2006). Culture. *Contexts, 5*(1), 43–44. https://doi.org/10.1525/ctx.2006.5.issue-1

Gutman, H. G. (1976). *The Black family in slavery and freedom, 1750–1925*. Blackwell.

Harvey, A. R., & Coleman, A. A. (1997). An Afrocentric program for African American males in the juvenile justice system. *Child Welfare, 76*, 197–211.

Harvey, A. R., & Rauch, J. B. (1997). A comprehensive Afrocentric rites of passage program for Black male adolescents. *Health & Social Work, 22*, 30–37. https://doi.org/10.1093/hsw/22.1.30

Hill, P. Jr. (1992). Coming of Age: African American Male Rites of Passage. Chicago: African American Images.

Johnson, V. E., & Carter, R. T. (2020). Black cultural strengths and psychosocial well-being: An empirical analysis with Black American adults. *Journal of Black Psychology, 46*(1), 55–89. https://doi.org/10.1177/0095798419889752

Karenga, M. (2008). *Kwanzaa: A celebration of family, community and culture*. University of Sankore Press.

Kuwornu-Adjaottor, J. E. T., Appiah, G., & Nartey, M. (2016). The philosophy behind some Adinkra symbols and their communicative values in Akan. *Philisophical Papers and Review, 7*(3), 22–33.

Laitin, D., & Weingast, B. R. (2006). An equilibrium alternative to the study of culture. *The Good Society, 15*(1), 15–20.

Madhubuti, H. R. (1991). *Black men: Obsolete, single, sangerous? Afikan American families in transition: Essays in discovery, solutions, and hope*. Third World Press.

McCashen, W. (2005). *The strengths approach: A strengths-based resource for sharing power and creating change*. St. Lukes Innovative Resources.

Men Healing Men and Communities Strategic Plan. (2015). Retrieved from https://www.memphis.edu/cayd/pdfs/mhmcn-strategic-plan.pdf

Mensah, A. (n.d.). *Rites of passage and initiation processes with Akan Culture*.

National Alliance on Mental Illness. (n.d.). Retrieved from https://namica.org/wp-content/uploads/2016/07/Breakout-Session-Outcomes.pdf

Nobles, W., Goodard, L., Gavil, W., & George, P. (1987). *The culture of drugs in the black community*. The Black Family Institute.

Potts, R. G. (2013). Right of passage is in prison settings: Interrupting rituals of mass Incarceration. *Black Child Journal: Special Edition*: Summer Edition 133–139.

Saleebey, D. (2002). *The strengths perspective in social work practice*. Allyn and Bacon.

Serpell, Z., Hayling, C. C., Stevenson, H., & Kern, L. (2009). Cultural considerations in the development of school- based interventions for African-American adolescent boys with emotional and behavioral disorders. *Journal of Negro Education, 78*(3), 321–332.

Snow, L. K. (2004). *The power of asset mapping: How your congregation can act on its gifts*. The Alban Institute.

Somé, M. P. (1993). *Ritual: Power, healing and community*. Swan/Raven.

Song, Y. (2009). Identity and duality. *Art Education, 62*(6), 19–24.

Stepteau-Watson, D., Watson, J., & Lawrence, S. (2014). Young African American Males in reentry: An Afrocentric cultural approach. *Journal of Human Behavior in the Social Environment, 24*(6).: Promotion of Young African American Male Health, 658–665. https://doi.org/10.1080/10911359.2014.922801

Wahler, E. A. (2012). Identifying and challenging social work student biases. *Social Work Education, 31*(8), 1058–1070.

Washington, G., Caldwell, L. D., Watson, J., & Lindsey, L. (2017). African American rites of passage interventions: A vehicle for utilizing African American male elders. *Journal of Human Behavior in the Social Environment, 24*(6), 658–655. https://doi.org/10.1080/1091135 9.2016.1266858

Whaley, A. L., & Noël, L. T. (2012). Sociocultural theories, academic achievement and African-American adolescents in a multicultural context: A review of the cultural compatibility perspective. *Journal of Negro Education, 81*(1), 25–38. https://doi.org/10.7709/jnegroeducation.81.1.0025

Jerry Watson, PhD, LCSW, MBA, is an assistant professor and coordinator of the Bachelor of Social Work program at the University of Memphis in Tennessee. Jerry taught sociology and psychology at DePaul University, group work at Aurora University in Chicago, and a variety of social work courses at the bachelor's, master's, and doctoral levels at Jackson State University, Mississippi Valley State University, the University of Mississippi, and Rust College. Jerry currently teaches and is the faculty lead at the University of Memphis for Social Work Practice in Community and Organizations. Dr. Watson is a scholar-activist and generalist practitioner. Jerry has over 50 years of combined experience in teaching, working in a variety of community clinical positions, and leading health and wellness programs and initiatives targeting African American men and boys. Dr. Watson's community experience and scholarship spans broadly across community topics including the following domains with a social justice lens: offender re-entry support, affordable housing, community organizing, business development, asset-based community development, cultural activism, youth and family wellness, crime and safety, community violence intervention and prevention, trauma-informed care, the "digital divide," race, culture, and poverty.

Gregory Washington, PhD, LCSW, is a professor in the School of Social Work at the University of Memphis, Tennessee. Washington is the Director of the Center for the Advancement of Youth Development, a Program Advisor for the Benjamin L. Hooks Institute for Social Change African American Male Initiative, and the current Director of the African American Male Academy at the University of Memphis. Dr. Washington works as a community clinical practitioner and has practiced as an individual, family and group therapist in Illinois, Georgia, Arkansas, and Tennessee. His research interests include culturally centered empowerment methods and the risk and protective factors associated with youth development. A major goal of his work is to identify and promote the use of innovative culturally centered group interventions that reduce risk for disparities in behavioral health and incarceration outcomes among young people of color.

Part III
Black Men in Research

Chapter 8
Asserting Voice: Navigating Service Delivery and Community Resources

Jennifer A. Wade-Berg

There is no denying that inequity exists within health care for black males. The chapters in this book attest to the nature of how these inequities manifest themselves and the impact they have on black men, their families, and the community in which they live. Upon understanding the complexity associated with these problems, black men and advocates seek to find solutions. This chapter explores and asserts that black men must use their individual and collective voice to not only improve upon the current healthcare delivery system but perhaps use new strategies aimed at creating community-based resources aimed at improving their health and well-being. The purpose of this chapter is to explore one such strategy – the utilization of nonprofit organizations and collaborative networks to create new service integration opportunities around health care for black men.

An Old Concept Revisited

Empowerment and conscious raising are not new concepts for the black community. Since the founding of America and with the beginning of slavery, blacks have been fighting for social, economic, and political equity and equality. Various strategies have been utilized over time to overcome these inequities and inequalities, including, but not limited to, nonviolent social action, political advocacy, and challenges to the court system. However, a strategy often overlooked, and the theme of this chapter, centers on the positioning of nonprofit organizations as supplemental service providers and conduits of change.

J. A. Wade-Berg (✉)
Department of Social Work and Human Services, Kennesaw State University, Atlanta, GA, USA
e-mail: jwadeber@kennesaw.edu

© The Author(s), under exclusive license to Springer Nature Switzerland AG 2022
Y. D. Dyson et al. (eds.), *Black Men's Health*,
https://doi.org/10.1007/978-3-031-04994-1_8

There are 27 types of nonprofit organizations as identified by the Internal Revenue Service (IRS) tax code. Nonprofit organizations make up what is deemed to be an important and recognizable economic sector. This distinction was made evident with the Commission on Private Philanthropy and Public Needs or the Filer Commission's findings (1973–1975). The Filer Commission noted that nonprofit organizations serve as initiators and developers of new ideas, public policies, and processes; supporters of minority, local, and foreign interests; and providers who supplement or direct provision of services to government, the citizenry, and/or for-profit organizations. Feiock and Jang (2003) also write about the importance of nonprofit organizations as supplemental providers of service, especially in health and human services.

According to the IRS, to be tax-exempt under section 501(c)(3) of the Internal Revenue Code, "an organization must be organized and operated exclusively for exempt purposes set forth in section 501(c)(3), and none of its earnings may inure to any private shareholder or individual. In addition, it may not be an action organization, i.e., it may not attempt to influence legislation as a substantial part of its activities, and it may not participate in any campaign activity for or against political candidates" (IRS, 2021). The types germane to this discussion are charitable (501c3) and general welfare (501c4) nonprofit organizations. The Internal Revenue Service classifies 501(c)4 organizations as general welfare or civic leagues. Organizations described in section 501(c)(3), other than testing for public safety organizations, are eligible to receive tax-deductible contributions in accordance with Code section 170. Contributions to 501(c)(4) organizations generally are not deductible as charitable contributions for federal income tax purposes.

One only needs to examine all major United States social movements to understand the importance of nonprofit organizations in changing the social, economic, and political landscape. For example, the United States Civil Rights Movement (1954–1968) was led by nonprofit organizations such as the Black Church, the National Urban League, the National Association for the Advancement of Colored People (NAACP), the Southern Christian Leadership Conference (SCLC), the Black Panther Party for Self-Defense, Student Nonviolent Coordinating Committee (SNCC), and Congress on Racial Equality (CORE). In 2021, the Black Lives Matter movement was led by nonprofit organizations such as Black Alliance for Just Immigration, Color of Change, the Movement for Black Lives, NAACP Legal Defense and Educational Fund, Inc., and UndocuBlack Network. Thus, it is not inconceivable that the black community turns to the idea of creating new networks or calls upon existing nonprofit organizations to address black men's health.

Service Integration: An Effective Solution to Raising Voice, Visibility, and Consciousness

To implement this idea, let us begin by understanding two basic ways that nonprofit organizations can work together, that is, collaboration and service integration.

Collaboration, as defined by O'Looney (1996, as cited by Wade-Berg & Robinson-Dooley, 2015), refers to the "generic process by which individuals and groups grow to be more positively interdependent and learn to coordinate their activities in ways that provide for synergistic benefits" (p. 121). While service integration is viewed to be a formal element of collaboration that can exist within four different models: service delivery or frontline-centered service integration; program-centered service delivery; policy-centered service integration; and organizationally centered service integration (Agranoff & Pattakos, 1979; Kagan, 1993; O'Looney 1996, as cited by Wade-Berg & Robinson-Dooley, 2015). Program-centered service integration alleviates problems in the service system infrastructure to provide for greater efficiency and effectiveness by improving the experiences of clients/customers. Experience benefits are in terms of an easy one-stop access to services and increased in personal services. Policy-centered service integration involves the engagement of the government in multiple activities to increase the efficiency of service delivery, including capacity building, priority setting, and system monitoring. Organizational-centered service integration involves the reorganization of governance structures, realignment of reward mechanisms personnel systems, and the reallocation of responsibilities within and across agencies. This concept is close to the idea of the development of a new service system.

While collaboration can provide an opportunity for nonprofit organizations to share resources while maintaining their individuality, it would be far better for organizational-centered service integration to occur to achieve higher impact and results when providing health care for black men. This type of service integration allows men to essentially utilize a one-stop shop for all things related to health. It also calls for organizations to remove barriers to address access issues and meet their clients in the community where they are. This idea is championed by the World Health Organization (WHO).

In a 2008 Technical Brief entitled Integrative Health Services, the WHO championed an overall definition for integrated health services as "[t]he management and delivery of health services so that clients receive a continuum of preventive and curative services, according to their needs over time and across different levels of the health system" (p. 1). It was their belief that this would solve for existing fragmentation that exists in the delivery of health care for black men. The brief goes on to explain that integration for the end user "means health care that is seamless, smooth, and easy to navigate. Users want a coordinated service which minimizes both the number of stages in an appointment and the number of separate visits required to a health facility. They want health workers to be aware of their health (not just one clinical aspect) and for the health workers from different levels of a system to communicate well. In short, clients want a continuity of care" (p. 5). For providers, senior managers, and policymakers, the WHO asserts that management, finance, and decision-making cannot be compartmentalized. Instead, close coordination along the lines of strategic alliances must be formed.

This concept is extremely complex to implement due to the tedious process and associated costs, for example, time, effort, resources, and organizational ego (O'Looney, 1994, as cited by Wade-Berg & Robinson-Dooley, 2015). Yet, research still suggests that this is still a beneficial solution because it can address the many problems that can exist due to service delivery fragmentation, fractured bureaucracy, and high transactional costs. When achieved successfully, one finds greater efficacy, effectiveness, and increased client sensitivity because: "(1) consumers are able to find everything they want because services are integrated and made available through [one stop] centers; (2) access to services is assured through programs being linked to one another; (3) a more comprehensive set of services is made available because of a more coordinated system of planning; (4) a better fit is made between consumers and community needs and the array of services made available because of more coordinated planning, information sharing, and pooling of agency funds; and (5) direct service staff becomes more knowledgeable of the entire array of services, and is less loyal to their own agency's need to retain clients, especially when these clients would be better served elsewhere" (O'Looney, 1993, as cited by Wade-Berg & Robinson-Dooley, 2015, p. 124).

Continuing the Dialogue

In 2010, the Office of Minority Health held a national dialogue entitled Effective Holistic Health for African Americans/Blacks in Washington, DC. The dialogue addressed specific concerns related to "addressing mental health, substance use/abuse, primary care, and the critically needed support services from a holistic health paradigm for Americans of African ancestry in the United States" (Davis et al., 2011, p.3). There are few service integration (and collaborative) only models focused on the care of Blacks and in particular with that of black males. What is prevalent are various organizations such as the Black Church; service-oriented non-profit organizations focused on the black community, such as historically black fraternities, 100 Black Men, etc; or the rise of single organizational models using an intentional philosophy of providing culturally specific and/or sensitive information, such as the Black Wellness Project and the African American Wellness Project. While these organizations certainly play a pivotal role in raising our consciousness, they must be coupled with direct service delivery designs that can offer direct services. Yet, these models are still too few (See Table 8.1). They are even more difficult to find when specifically looking for services focused on black health care.

Thus, in this post-COVID and George Floyd era, more attention is being focused on health inequity. Now is the time for community stakeholders to come together to place new models into practice. When creating these service integrative models, the recommendations by the Office of Minority Health should be revisited (See Table 8.2).

Intentional service delivery systems/designs of integrated health services for black men must be created in their communities that also infuse other unique social and economic support services based on population needs for real change to occur, like the Dimock Center

Table 8.1 Examples of integrated health care

Organization	Mission	Services	Service integration	Website
The Dimock Center	"With a mission to heal and uplift individuals and families, we endeavor to redefine the model of a healthy community by creating equitable access to comprehensive health care and education."	(a) Health center (e.g., eye, dental, adult primary care, pharmacy), (b) child and family development services (e.g., head start, early intervention), and (c) behavioral health services (e.g., emergency shelter, counseling and addiction, residential, detox center)	The Center integrates education, health care, housing.	www.dimock.org
School-based health initiatives		Varies with each school. Common services: Breakfast/food services during holiday and summer breaks, immunizations, oral care, mental or behavioral health coupled with K-12 education	Integration of education and healthcare services, e.g., school-based health alliance	Sbh4all.org

Table 8.2 Consensus statements by the Office of Minority Health (Davis et al., 2011)

1. A long-term response to health disparities in African American communities has been the development of informal or practice-based evidence as well as the use of healers. For behavioral health care and related problems, African Americans often seek services from their houses of worship. However, there is a need to assess Pathways to Integrated Health Care: Strategies for African American Communities and Organizations. These interventions determine the effectiveness of their outcomes and how the interventions can become evidence-based practices.

2. Reductions in disparities are partially dependent on the quality, quantity, and skills of the health and behavioral health workforce and the type of integrated care applied. There is a need for a more diverse workforce that utilizes culturally and linguistically proficient and competent interventions that are developed within African American communities in addition to those that may also involve adaptations of evidence-based practices from other communities.

3. There is a pressing need to develop and measure a core set of practice standards and criteria that focus on holistic health, wellness, and community-based standards.

4. A significant number of health and behavioral health conditions in African American communities co-morbid with other socio-economic conditions. These co-occurring conditions include substance disorders, severe mental illness, HIV/AIDS, poverty, diabetes, heart disease, low income, unemployment, and homelessness as examples. The presence of multiple conditions increases overall health risks, stigma, costs, and health outcomes.

Source: https://www.minorityhealth.hhs.gov/Assets/pdf/Checked/1/PathwaystoIntegratedHealthCareStrategiesforAfricanAmericans.pdf

Summary

Navigating the health care system for black males can be difficult and often challenging given the lack of specificity and attention paid to the cultural nuances associated with health services for this population. This chapter underscores the inequity that exists within health care for black males by focusing on the service delivery system. Using a model of integrated health care delivery facilitated by community-based nonprofit organizations as an intermediary, black physicians, social workers, and supporting human service workers are finding ways to address the inequity that exists in the delivery of service. These integrated health care models are addressing the inequity gap by providing culturally relevant and responsive systems of care for black men (and their families).

Discussion Questions
1. Why are nonprofit organizations important to the service delivery system for the health care of black males?
2. What are the political, social, and economic challenges that black men and advocates meet when trying to create new service delivery strategies? How can one overcome them?
3. Why are organizations resistant to the idea of service integration?

Exercises
1. Identify a local community and create an asset map that identifies organizations and resources for meeting the health needs of black men. Identify the existence of gaps and propose new strategies and resources? Is there a space to reconfigure and create a new service delivery system?
2. Identify a local community and a health issue that black men experience. Create a new integrated service integration model to meet these needs.

Glossary of Terms and Concepts
Community-Based Organization (CBO): Deriving its roots from community social work, a community-based organization means a public or private nonprofit organization of demonstrated effectiveness that: (1) is representative of a community or significant segments of a community and (2) provides educational or related services to individuals in the community.

Integrated Health Services: The management and delivery of health services so that clients receive a continuum of preventive and curative services, according to their needs over time and across different levels of the health system (World Health Organization, 2008).

Nonprofit Charitable Organization: A business that has been granted tax-exempt status by the Internal Revenue Service and is organized exclusively for the purposes of furthering religious, scientific, charitable, educational, literary, public safety, or cruelty-prevention causes or purposes. These organizational types must also prohibit participating in political campaigns on behalf of any candidate or making expenditures for political purposes and must dedicate their assets to meet their exempt purpose in their organizing documents. The earnings must not inure benefit to any private shareholder or individual. Donors to these types of organizations may exercise a tax deduction on income tax. These organizations fall under the 501c3 Internal Revenue Tax Code. See www.irs.gov for a more complete discussion of tax implications.

Nonprofit Social Welfare Organization: An organization that has been granted tax-exempt status by the Internal Revenue Service and is organized exclusively to promote social welfare. The earnings must not inure benefit to any private shareholder or individual. These organizations enjoy greater lobbying benefits, and donors may not exercise a tax deduction. These organizations fall under the 501c4 Internal Revenue Tax Code. See www.irs.gov for a more complete discussion of tax implications.

References

Davis, K., & United States Department of Health and Human Services Office of Minority Health. (2011). *Pathways to integrated health: Strategies for African American communities and organizations*. Available at: https://www.minorityhealth.hhs.gov/Assets/pdf/Checked/1/PathwaystoIntegratedHealthCareStrategiesforAfricanAmericans.pdf

Feiock, R. C., & Jang, H. (2003). *The role of nonprofits in delivery of local services*. A paper presented at the National Public Management Research Association Meeting and supported by a grant from the Aspen Institute Nonprofit Research Fund. Available at: https://citeseerx.ist.psu.edu/viewdoc/download?doi=10.1.1.614.4721&rep=rep1&type=pdf

Internal Revenue Service (IRS). (2021). *Exemption requirements – 501(c)(3) organizations*. https://www.irs.gov/charities-non-profits/charitable-organizations/exemption-requirements-501c3-organizations

Wade-Berg, J. A., & Robinson-Dooley, V. (2015). Perceptions of collaboration and service integration as strategic alternatives: An examination of social service nonprofit organizations in the late 1990s. *Journal of Public Management & Social Policy, 20*(2), Article 2. Available at: http://digitalscholarship.tsu.edu/jpmsp/vol20/iss2/2

World Health Organization (2008) *Integrated health services-what and why?* (A technical brief no. 1). https://www.who.int/healthsystems/service_delivery_techbrief1.pdf

Jennifer A. Wade-Berg, PhD, CNP, is Associate Professor of Human Services and Campus Executive Director of the Nonprofit Leadership Alliance Certificate Program. She also serves as Assistant Dean of Student Success in the Wellstar College of Health and Human Services at Kennesaw State University in Kennesaw, Georgia. She received a Bachelor of Arts in Government from Wesleyan University (Connecticut), and master's and doctoral degrees in Public Administration from the University of Georgia. Dr. Wade-Berg has received more than $6 million in private foundation, federal and internal institutional funding. Her teaching emphasis is nonprofit management and research interests include cultural competence, sports philanthropy, student success (recruitment, retention and progression to graduation), and nonprofit management.

Chapter 9
"The Talk" Revisited: Expanding the Conversation with Black Males in Trauma

Kara Beckett

While racially charged incidents are not a new phenomenon, the proliferation of raw images and videos depicting police brutality, and in many cases showing police officers killing unarmed Black men, women, and children via the Internet, is. Fatal incidents, including deadly shootings of unarmed Black men by police officers, have inundated the media over the past 9 years creating increased public awareness domestically and internationally. High-profile cases such as George Floyd, Michael Brown, Eric Garner, Tamir Rice, Walter Scott, and Philando Castile, and the vigilante cases of Trayvon Martin and Ahmaud Arbery, sparked a national conversation on racism and the relationship between law enforcement and the Black community.

The varied cases and subsequent global response raises consciousness and brings into focus the phenomenological experience of a Black body and theorizing it as an object; undervalued, less than, and not equal to the human race. The lack of punishment to police officers, even with seemingly hard-core evidence, causes social justice advocates to think strategically about how to address this problem. More specifically, it has created a social media–specific civil rights moment bringing to life the Black Lives Matter (BLM) movement.

Black men are disproportionately affected by police violence. According to a recent study in the Proceedings of the National Academies of Sciences, Black men face a one in 1000 chance of having a fatal encounter with the police (Edwards et al., 2019). Police violence is the seventh leading cause of death for Black men aged 25–29 years (Edwards et al., 2019). The reality of possible death at the hands of law enforcement and everyday citizens, coupled with the persistent exposure to racial discrimination, can lead to psychological symptoms, including hypervigilance, anxiety, and depression.

K. Beckett (✉)
Barbara Solomon School of Social Work, Walden University, Minneapolis, MN, USA
e-mail: kara.beckett@mail.waldenu.edu

© The Author(s), under exclusive license to Springer Nature Switzerland AG 2022
Y. D. Dyson et al. (eds.), *Black Men's Health*,
https://doi.org/10.1007/978-3-031-04994-1_9

These factors lead to the overarching theme of this chapter: How can social work practitioners address the deleterious effects of racial trauma on Black men? Examining this question requires clinicians to be aware of the impact and be prepared to address racial trauma and racial discrimination with Black men in their ongoing clinical work. This chapter explores the mental health effects of racial trauma among Black men during this crucial time in history when the American Medical Association (AMA) and the Centers for Disease Control and Prevention (CDC) have both declared racism a public health threat (O'Reilly, 2020; CDC, 2021). Selected details from the case of Kevin highlight his experience with racial trauma and explore the mental health effects of racism. Revisiting the concept of "the talk," initially conceptualized as a conversation between Black parents and their children about race and racism and how to arrive back home safely and alive when stopped by the police and now applying it through the lens of engaging in difficult but necessary dialogue with Black men is necessary.

While this chapter is not intended for the sole purpose of an in-depth history lesson on the origination of the concepts of race, racism, and racial discrimination, it is necessary to define its meaning as it relates to this chapter. Racism is born out of the concept of race, a social construct designed to categorize and describe differences among people "...in the way we now understand ethnicity or natural identity" (Clair & Denis, 2015, para. 3). Most social scientists have dismissed the notion of race as a biological variable, but it continues to have a tremendous impact on the structure of society. Camara Jones, MD, Research Director on Social Determinants of Health and Equity, CDC, describes the impervious nature of race and further elaborates on the concept of race as:

> ...a social classification based on phenotype, that governs the distribution of risks and opportunities in our race-conscious society. Although ethnicity reflects cultural heritage, race measures a societally imposed identity and consequent exposure to the societal constraints associated with that particular identity. (Jones, 2000, p. 300)

As structured, the classification system of race is a hierarchy consisting of bodies of varying colors, with a level of worth and importance given to each. This notion of race makes racism possible. Racism is fundamentally a "system of advantage based on race" (Tatum, 2017, p. 87) that favors whiteness and can be expressed actively or passively. Wijeysinghe, Griffin, and Love (1997) describe racism as:

> The systemic subordination of members of targeted racial groups who have relatively little social power in the United States (Blacks, Latino/as, Native Americans, and Asians), by the members of the agent racial group who have relatively more social power (Whites). This subordination is supported by the actions of individuals, cultural norms and values, and the institutional structures and practices of society. (pp. 88–89)

Racial discrimination, in its simplest terms, is unequal treatment against a person based on their race or ethnic background.

Mental Health Effects of Racism

Over the past 10 years, there has been increased research on Black men and mental health. Because the landscape of mental illness is changing, as well as the factors that affect the mental health of Black men, it is imperative that clinicians are knowledgeable and can apply this knowledge to practice. Research has documented the harmful effects of racial discrimination on the mental health of Black Americans and the correlation to increased depressive symptoms and poorer health outcomes (Brondolo et al., 2009; Clark et al., 1999).

Depression is the number one disability affecting 264 million people worldwide (WHO, 2020). Psychosocial stressors, biochemical factors, and genetics are all risk factors, thus making anyone susceptible. While the overall prevalence of major depression for Black men is lower than for White men, it is often left untreated and chronic in nature, leading to more severe consequences (Williams et al., 2007). One such consequence is the feeling of hopelessness and helplessness, often experienced with depression, which can lead to suicide. Suicide is the third leading cause of death in Black men aged 25–34 years (NIMH, 2021). It is important to note thàt the suicide mortality rate of Black men has increased at a higher rate than compared to White men from the years 2000–2014 (Pathak, 2018).

A discussion about Black men and mental health should include the adverse life experiences faced that lead to injurious mental health outcomes. Higher rates of poverty, mortality, and unemployment and increased exposure to racial discrimination and perceived discrimination require further examination (Watkins et al., 2006). Specifically, the more recent occurrences of racial profiling by everyday White citizens – Driving While Black (DWB), walking in your neighborhood, shopping while Black, and being Black in your own home – widens the lens of the effects of racism on Black men's mental health. It reinforces the negative stereotypes held throughout history and the extensive research suggesting that Black men are "viewed as the prototypical criminal" (Chaney & Robertson, 2013, p. 482). These racialized incidents are common occurrences and have created an enhanced concern for safety and well-being that is unique to Black men.

The addition of police brutality and the fatal shootings by police officers, disproportionately affecting Black men, adds another layer of factors that adversely affect mental health. The shooting death of Michael Brown and his body laying on the ground for more than four hours and the murder of George Floyd, both by police officers, gave witnesses, community members, and other people who were on the scene the chance to take photos and videos with their smartphones and immediately upload them to various social media websites. The images circulated on the Internet at record speed, before the first news report aired. The anger that ensued over the disregard of a Black body is evident, regardless of the details. It is reminiscent of a longstanding history of discrimination, unfair and improper treatment, and numerous cases that did not receive national attention.

Racial Trauma: The Case of Kevin[1]

> Silence. A space we frequented, but this time a minute felt like an eternity. Kevin held his head in his hands, rocking back and forth while taking sporadic deep breaths. He called to come in a week earlier than our next scheduled session. I knew the urgency of the moment. "When is it going to stop? I can't get it out of my head. I close my eyes and all I see is that white officer kneeling on his neck. I open my eyes, look at the TV and my social media feed, and I see it over and over again."

Kevin, a 26-year-old Black man, has been in therapy for 6 months. He sought treatment after encouragement from close friends due to feelings of anger, anxiety, and depression stemming from workplace discrimination. Upon conducting the assessment, Kevin disclosed that his feelings of depression and anxiety did not just start from issues at work, but have been building over time. His intense emotions stemmed from the racism and racial discrimination he endured over the years from childhood to the present.

Kevin disclosed a history of harassment by police officers starting at the age of 12 years old. He witnessed his childhood friend being aggressively handled by the police and experienced microaggressions and racial discrimination while in college, and subsequently on his job. Additionally, Kevin is emotionally affected by countless videos displayed and viewed repeatedly on social media of Black men and women killed by law enforcement, such as Breonna Taylor and George Floyd. The intensity of these feelings, coupled with the difficulty of managing them, impacts his daily functioning.

Kevin's narrative of negative interactions with police officers is similar to the experience of many Black men growing up, especially those residing in an urban area. When the police drove by his home, he was continuously approached and "bothered" by police officers. Even when he felt he was not engaged in behaviors that one would deem illegal, the result was the same. It was a common occurrence, even though he was a child. In the article, "The Essence of Innocence: Consequences of Dehumanizing Black Children" (2014), Goff et al. examined whether Black boys were given the same protections in childhood equal to their peers. Using a novel scale created to measure innocence, student participants selected from a large university completed the questionnaire to measure how innocent children were in general without respect to race and how innocent Black and White children were (Goff et al., 2014). In general, the results showed that all children, regardless of race, are innocent from ages 0–9. However, the perception of innocence had different results between the races in children over age 10 worth noting. Black children are perceived as, "...significantly less innocent than other children at every age group, beginning at the age of 10" (p. 529). An interesting dynamic occurred where the perceived innocence of black children in the age group 10–13 years "...was equivalent to that of non-Black children age 14–17, and the perceived innocence of Black children age 14–17 was equivalent to that of non-Black adults age 18–21" (p. 529),

---

[1] All names and identifying factors in the chapter have been changed for client confidentiality.

thus substantiating that Black children are viewed as older in advance of their stated age, thus leading to widespread implications. Research has shown that Black youth are stopped, questioned, and arrested at higher rates than white youth (Epp et al., 2014).

> I just remember being nervous…each time I would see one of them. It became normal, but I didn't feel normal. I would sweat, my heart raced…I even felt like I was gonna pass out. I couldn't run away though, it would make it seem like I did something wrong when all I was doing was playing with my friends, doing kid stuff. It was worse after my friend was slammed on the ground. Sometimes I think about that over and over again, especially when I'm driving and see a cop behind me. They can do whatever because I'm Black. That's how I have to live my life and I'll never forget that.

Kevin is experiencing hyperarousal, anxiety, and intrusive thoughts as a result of his negative interaction with police officers. He is fearful of future interactions because a higher level of consciousness exists where a seemingly simple situation could go awry based on previous personal experience or witnessing the incidents of others. The impact of dashcams and cell phone recordings has brought awareness to a prevailing issue. However, because there has not been significant punishment for the numerous incidents of police brutality and deaths, he feels vulnerable and defeated, and it fosters the belief that his life does not matter. "When police perpetrate violence, this belief is shattered as the police are no longer protectors but rather the central threat that needs to be addressed" (DeVylder et al., 2020, p. 4). This causes Kevin to avoid, to the extent possible, any contact with law enforcement. The sense of powerlessness is overwhelming for him.

Kevin's emotional reaction to his experiences fits within the conceptualization of trauma. The American Psychiatric Association (2013) defines a traumatic event as:

> …exposure to actual or threatened death, serious injury, or sexual violence and can take place in one or more of the following ways: (1) directly experiencing the traumatic event(s), (2) witnessing, in person, the event(s) as it occurred to others, (3) learning that the traumatic event(s) occurred to a close family member or close friend and in cases of actual/threatened death of a friend or family member the event(s) must have been violent or accidental, and (4) experiencing repeated or extreme exposure to aversive details of the traumatic event(s). (p. 271)

Specifically, Kevin's lived experience is indicative of racial trauma. Racial trauma is trauma due to experiences of racism, either real or perceived. It can transpire from one specific event or be the result of an accumulation of encounters, including subtle forms like microaggressions. This form of discrimination can be more harmful than overt and explicit displays of racism. Racial trauma is different from other forms of trauma because "victims are targeted solely on the basis of their race and ethnicity" (Comas-Diaz, 2016, p. 251). Carter (2007) explains that "race-based events are often not physical, they occur across the life span, and they usually reoccur in different situations and contexts" (p. 34). The exposure is constant and enduring, thereby causing psychological wounds. The culmination of events from chronic exposure to racism, either directly or vicariously, can be traumatizing.

Digital Media and Racism

The convergence of digital media and racism has created a new era of visualizing traumatic events in real time. These encounters are difficult to avoid on the Internet as race and racism are persistent and pervasive, especially how it plays out on social networking sites (SNS) (Daniels, 2013). For Kevin, witnessing continuous acts of police brutality and killing of Black men in the media elicits terror and dread when he sees a police officer. The research is scant on the psychological impact of Black men who "view, read, or hear of the killings of unarmed Black men via various media outlets" (Lipscomb et al., 2019, p. 11). Lipscomb and his research team added to this body of knowledge with a phenomenological qualitative research study investigating how 62 young adult Black men experienced the 2018 fatal shooting of Stephon Clark in California (Lipscomb et al., 2019). Although the results are not generalizable,

> The narratives highlight pain among Black men who are forced to choose their poison: death by a fear-fragility induced bullet or the psychological anguish that inevitably comes from not being able to simply live and be. Black males have been subjected to prove the value of their psychological and emotional existence each day, no matter what privileges Black males may carry from being male. (p. 16)

While her research did not focus on Black men, Dr. Pam Ramsden at the University of Bradford led a study on the long-term effects of stress, anxiety, and PTSD from viewing graphic images on social media (Hope, 2015). In her study of 189 participants, Ramsden uses PTSD clinical assessments, a vicarious trauma assessment, and a questionnaire about violent events seen on social media or the Internet (2015). Ramsden's preliminary results show that 22% scored high on the PTSD clinical measures assessment and were affected by the media events shown (2015). The participants did not have a prior history of trauma.

Implications for Practice and Treatment

While there are psychosocial factors that prevent young Black men from seeking medical care, this too exists in the realm of mental health. Historically, Black men have underutilized mental health treatment due to reasons including "racism and discrimination; mistrust of health care providers; misdiagnosis and clinician bias; and use of informal support networks" (Hankerson et al., 2015, p. 2). There is also a stigma surrounding mental health in the Black community thus creating treatment hesitancy. The longer mental illness is untreated, the greater risk for poorer outcomes.

Concerning Black men, issues of racial discrimination and inequality are prevalent in daily interactions on an individual or micro level, as well as a macro level, through agencies and organizations. It is equally important to recognize "...racist incidents as potentially traumatizing stressors" (Bryant-Davis & Ocampo, 2006,

p. 4). Conceptualizing treatment through a trauma lens can assist with understanding symptoms such as hypervigilance, avoidance, intense fear, and distress. If there is an unawareness, minimization, or denial of this experience, it can disrupt the therapeutic alliance, thus providing a disservice to the client (Brown et al., 2013).

As a clinician, self-awareness is necessary, specifically relating to understanding your own racial identity (Bryant-Davis & Ocampo, 2006). Unconscious biases, perceptions, and ideologies can directly influence engagement, interactions, and developing a trusting relationship with a client. In the article "Clinical Social Work's Contribution to a Social Justice Perspective," Swenson (1998) explores a variety of theories and practices that social justice can be applied to clinical social work. Reflexivity is an ongoing process of professional development utilized to focus attention on one's values, thoughts, actions, and biases. Reflexivity in social justice "…requires that practitioners pay careful attention to their own experiences of oppression and of privilege or domination" (p. 532). Developing a keen awareness of personal beliefs, opinions, and behaviors impacts the helping profession and how change is affected. Becoming aware of the lack of knowledge while working with clients from various populations is uncovered through the practice of being self-reflexive. Self-awareness of personal experiences and understanding the view from a client's perspective as one in a position of power is a starting point.

Social workers are educated on the importance of cultural competence and have an ethical responsibility to be knowledgeable about issues concerning diverse populations, as per the National Association of Social Workers (NASW) Code of Ethics:

> (a) Social workers should understand culture and its function in human behavior and society, recognizing the strengths that exist in all cultures. (b) Social workers should have a knowledge base of their clients' cultures and be able to demonstrate competence in the provision of services that are sensitive to clients' cultures and to differences among people and cultural groups. (c) Social workers should obtain education about and seek to understand the nature of social diversity and oppression with respect to race, ethnicity, national origin, color, sex, sexual orientation, gender identity or expression, age, marital status, political belief, religion, immigration status, and mental or physical ability. (d) Social workers should obtain education about and demonstrate understanding of the nature of social diversity and oppression with respect to race, ethnicity, national origin, color, sex, sexual orientation, gender identity or expression, age, marital status, political belief, religion, immigration status, and mental or physical ability. (NASW, 2017, Section 1.05 Cultural Competence)

Understanding the history of oppression in marginalized populations and the impact of racist incidents, especially in the current climate, is imperative as it can foster trust in the therapeutic relationship. Being able to identify how a client can face discrimination is paramount as these experiences shape a person's life. "The pain expressed by Black men must be understood within a context of an historical narrative of marginality and the psychosocial consequences of an oppressive past" (Lipscomb et al., 2019, p. 12). Social justice work in clinical social work "…means profound appreciation for a client's strengths, contexts, and resources" (Swenson, 1998, p. 534). Empowering a client and recognizing personal biases that can impact the therapeutic relationship is a step in creating a healthy client/therapist relationship.

Intersectionality Theory; the Criss-Cross of Social Identities, Social Systems, and Social Problems

Viewing a person through a narrow lens and only taking into account oppression as it relates to race is a singular approach to the multidimensional and complex social identities that make up a person. To fully understand the identity of a person, it is necessary to factor in the multidimensional aspects that intersect and impact a life. When considering race and the inevitable effects of racism, it is important to consider gender roles as negative connotations are associated with each identity. For example, racial profiling with Black men is ubiquitous. Being followed, stopped, questioned, and/or wrongfully accused for seemingly illegitimate reasons – by police officers, in retail stores, and in other spaces, is almost expected, especially in this current climate. Additionally, the portrayal of Black men in the media as dangerous and a threat to others contributes to negative thoughts and subsequent actions by authority figures and everyday citizens.

Kimberlé Crenshaw, JD, Professor of Law at UCLA, developed the concept of intersectionality theory in 1989 to address the complexity of discrimination and how it can be experienced in a multitude of ways. In essence, intersectionality is a sociological theory demonstrating how an individual can face discrimination in multiple ways when their identities overlap in several subordinate groups, such as race, age, gender, ethnicity, class, and other characteristics. To fully understand the dynamics of oppressed groups, one must examine the societal structures and processes that work simultaneously. Utilizing the frame of intersectionality theory helps to give a better understanding of the power relations at play and to ensure that the challenges of people who encompass multiple minority identities are not overlooked.

In a clinical setting, knowing how to extract the pertinent information while remaining engaged with the client as they tell their story is essential in the therapeutic relationship. Bracketing, or being subjective while eliminating objectivity, as well as the need/desire to label based on symptomology, is not always an easy task, as it requires a clinician to filter their mental models, theoretical frameworks, experiences, and perceptions about how the world works. Starting where the client is can best account for bracketing, because to do this, assumptions have to be set aside. Although clinicians assist clients with maneuvering through their stories to get to the root of the issue, it is important to listen to and process the lived experience that is crucial to treatment. Clinicians who engage in systematic reflection of practice, "…in particular their experiences of racism and oppression… can serve as a document of changing experiences and attitudes about racism over a professional life span" (Swenson, 1998, p. 532), leading to a more phenomenological approach in psychotherapy.

As clinicians, it is important to listen to what words mean and how they are experienced. In broadening the view of this statement and how it applies to the helping profession, one must be cautious on labeling, pathologizing behaviors, and making decisions on what is "normal" or not. According to Lewis-Fernández (2013, as cited in Cummings, 2015), a cultural psychiatrist from Columbia University who was the co-chair of the Gender and Cross-Cultural Issues Study Group for the *Diagnostic and Statistical Manual of Mental Disorders, Fifth Edition* (DSM-5):

> Each illness has to be assessed in its own right and both the practitioner's expertise and epistemological assumptions and the individual's understanding of the illness should apply. That is, the clinician must not only draw from diagnostic experience, available categories of illness, and the various dimensions along which aspects of the illness may range, but also recognize and try to understand each individual's anomalous experience. (para 6)

The DSM-5 does not take into account the context of one's situation as it is a manualized method that classifies symptomology to determine a diagnosis. As a context-dependent profession, a client is assessed based on the context of their lived experience. The subtle clues given through their narrative on what flourishing looks like for any particular client can easily be missed when it is only observed through the lens of society and what the leading authorities define as what "normal" is and should look like. Clients are often reduced to their symptomology, without a full understanding that symptoms serve a purpose. Sometimes it is difficult to press the pause button and forego looking at symptomology to then classifying it as a pathology, instead of sitting with what the experience is for a client, through their lens.

Working with Black men includes that there is a likelihood of having a negative experience due to their race. Therefore, it is important to assess for any racial trauma when exploring trauma history and be "mindful of the various ways in which this trauma may show up in the lives of Black males (i.e., anger, sadness, avoidance, dissociation and hypervigilance)" (Lipscomb et al., 2019, p. 16). Questions should include if the client has had a negative interaction or has been treated differently due to their race or cultural background and if they have witnessed a person being treated discriminatorily due to their race (Bryant-Davis and Ocampo, 2006). If racial incidents are disclosed, responding with empathy and support is necessary. Obtaining more detailed information about the incident(s), including feelings and thoughts of the experience, as well as the coping strategies used to mitigate the effects is essential. Special attention should be paid to any symptoms indicative of PTSD.

Summary

This particular moment of deepening racial division and differentiation requires clinicians to rethink and revise their work with Black men. Understanding the lived experience with racial discrimination and its current impact is paramount as these experiences shape a person's life. The narrative is an important component and can be seen as therapeutic and transformative. It can also provide a peek into the life of a person, their symptomology, and how it affects them. In essence, it emphasizes their account. The key is accepting and respecting what is disclosed without trying to conform it to what clinicians think it should be.

A clarion call exists for shifting perspectives, including moving from the societal viewpoint of Black men being perceived as criminals and dangerous, understanding racial trauma and the potential impact on their mental health, and giving voice to their lived experience. The therapeutic alliance, acceptance, and being open to the client's world and all that it entails decrease the chance of being treated as a symptom and more like a human being.

Racism, digital media, and the struggle to protect the Black body are factors that impact Black men and their mental health. Establishing a safe environment with trust, collaboration, and connection becomes paramount. Empowering a client and being aware of biases that can impact the therapeutic relationship is a step in creating a healthy client/therapist relationship. By engaging students and other mental health professionals who work with Black men in a therapeutic setting, it is the hope that this chapter serves as the start of a conversation, not the end.

Discussion Questions

1. The DSM-5 does not take into account racial trauma in PTSD. How might this affect treatment?
2. What therapeutic interventions are useful in working with Black men who suffer from racial trauma?
3. Why is it necessary to "bracket?" How would this help in the case of Kevin?

Exercises

1. Self-care can prove difficult with the onslaught of graphic images/videos of racial incidents and working with Black men who are seeking treatment for racial trauma. The intense exposure to traumatic events can lead to vicarious trauma. How would you implement a self-care regiment for yourself?
2. Write up a short case vignette of a Black male client you have personally worked with or from another case you may be familiar with. What questions would you ask under trauma history, specifically assessing for racial trauma?
3. Page 12 states, "Unconscious biases, perceptions, and ideologies can directly influence engagement, interactions, and developing a trusting relationship with a client." How can you become self-aware of your personal beliefs, and opinions? After reading this chapter, what are the next steps you can take to further your knowledge and understanding about working with Black men and their specialized needs?

Glossary of Terms and Concepts

Intersectionality theory: A sociological theory demonstrating how an individual can face discrimination in multiple ways when their identities overlap in several subordinate groups, such as race, age, gender, ethnicity, class, and other characteristics.

Microaggressions: Subtle slights that communicate bias directed to people of color and other marginalized populations.

Phenomenological experience: The subjective or lived experience of a person.

Racial discrimination: Unequal treatment against a person based on their race or ethnic background.

Racial trauma: Trauma due to experiences of racism, either real or perceived. It can transpire from one specific event or be the result of an accumulation of encounters, including subtle forms like microaggressions.

Reflexivity: It is an ongoing process of professional development utilized to focus attention on one's values, thoughts, actions, and biases.

Vicarious trauma: Indirect exposure to trauma occurring after repeatedly hearing clients recount traumatic events. As a result, the clinician can experience trauma symptoms and it can alter their worldview.

References

American Psychiatric Association. (2013). *Diagnostic and statistical manual of mental disorders* (5th ed.). Author.

Brondolo, E., Ver Halen, N. B., Pencille, M., Beatty, D., & Contrada, R. J. (2009). Coping with racism: A selective review of the literature and a theoretical and methodological critique. *Journal of Behavioral Medicine, 32*(1), 64–88.

Brown, D. L., Blackmon, S. K., Schumacher, K., & Urbanski, B. (2013). Exploring clinicians attitudes toward the incorporation of racial socialization in psychotherapy. *Journal of Black Psychology, 39*(6), 507–531.

Bryant-Davis, T., & Ocampo, C. (2006). A therapeutic approach to the treatment of racist-incident-based trauma. *Journal of Emotional Abuse, 6*(4), 1–22.

Carter, R. T. (2007). Racism and psychological and emotional injury: Recognizing and assessing race-based traumatic stress. *The Counseling Psychologist, 35*(1), 13–105.

Centers for Disease Control and Prevention. (2021, April 8). *Media statement from CDC Director Rochelle P. Walensky, MD, MPH, on racism and health.* https://www.cdc.gov/media/releases/2021/s0408-racism-health.html

Chaney, C., & Robertson, R. V. (2013). Racism and police brutality in America. *Journal of African American Studies, 17*(4), 480–505.

Clair, M., & Denis, J. (2015). *Sociology of racism.* Retrieved April 3, 2016, from http://scholar.harvard.edu/files/matthewclair/files/sociology_of_racism_clairandenis_2015.pdf

Clark, R., Anderson, N. B., Clark, V. R., & Williams, D. R. (1999). Racism as a stressor for African Americans: A biopsychosocial model. *American Psychologist, 54*(10), 805.

Comas-Díaz, L. (2016). Racial trauma recovery: A race-informed therapeutic approach to racial wounds. In A. N. Alvarez, C. T. H. Liang, & H. A. Neville (Eds.), *The cost of racism for people of color: Contextualizing experiences of discrimination* (pp. 249–272). American Psychological Association. https://doi.org/10.1037/14852-012

Cummings, C. (2015, February 13). *DSM-5 on culture: A significant advance.* Retrieved from https://thefpr.org/dsm-5-on-culture-a-significant-advance/

Daniels, J. (2013). Race and racism in Internet studies: A review and critique. *New Media & Society, 15*(5), 695–719.

DeVylder, J., Fedina, L., & Link, B. (2020). Impact of police violence on mental health: A theoretical framework. *American Journal of Public Health, 110*(11), 1704–1710.

Edwards, F., Lee, H., & Esposito, M. (2019). Risk of being killed by police use of force in the United States by age, race–ethnicity, and sex. *Proceedings of the National Academy of Sciences, 116*(34), 16793–16798.

Epp, C. R., Maynard-Moody, S., & Haider-Markel, D. P. (2014). *Pulled over: How police stops define race and citizenship.* University of Chicago Press.

Goff, P. A., Jackson, M. C., Di Leone, B. A. L., Culotta, C. M., & DiTomasso, N. A. (2014). The essence of innocence: Consequences of dehumanizing Black children. *Journal of Personality and Social Psychology, 106*(4), 526.

Hankerson, S. H., Suite, D., & Bailey, R. K. (2015). Treatment disparities among African American men with depression: Implications for clinical practice. *Journal of Health Care for the Poor and Underserved, 26*(1), 21.

Hope, J. (2015, May 7). *Online videos can cause post-traumatic stress disorder: One in five who view violent news events have lasting effects.* Retrieved from http://www.dailymail.co.uk/health/article-3071103/Online-videos-cause-post-traumatic-stress-disorder.html

Jones, C. P. (2000). Levels of racism: A theoretic framework and a gardener's tale. *American Journal of Public Health, 90*(8), 1212.

Lipscomb, A. E., Emeka, M., Bracy, I., Stevenson, V., Lira, A., Gomez, Y. B., & Riggins, J. (2019). Black male hunting! A phenomenological study exploring the secondary impact of police induced trauma on the Black man's psyche in the United States. *Journal of Sociology, 7*(1), 11–18.

National Association of Social Workers. (2017). *NASW code of ethics.* Retrieved from https://www.socialworkers.org/About/Ethics/Code-of-Ethics/Code-of-Ethics-English

National Institute of Mental Health. (2021, January). *Suicide.* https://www.nimh.nih.gov/health/statistics/suicide

O'Reilly, K. (2020, November 16). *AMA: Racism is a threat to public health.* American Medical Association. https://www.ama-assn.org/delivering-care/health-equity/ama-racism-threat-public-health

Pathak, E. B. (2018). Mortality among Black men in the USA. *Journal of Racial and Ethnic Health Disparities, 5*(1), 50–61.

Swenson, C. R. (1998). Clinical social work's contribution to a social justice perspective. *Social Work, 43*(6), 527–537.

Tatum, B. D. (2017). *"Why are all the Black kids sitting together in the cafeteria?" And other conversations about race.* Basic Books.

Watkins, D. C., Green, B. L., Rivers, B. M., & Rowell, K. L. (2006). Depression and Black men: Implications for future research. *Journal of Men's Health and Gender, 3*(3), 227–235.

Wijeysinghe, C. L., Griffin, P., & Love, B. (1997). Racism curriculum design. In M. Adams, L. A. Bell, & P. Griffin (Eds.), *Teaching for diversity and social justice: A sourcebook* (1st ed., pp. 82–109). Routledge.

Williams, D. R., Gonzalez, H. M., Neighbors, H., Nesse, R., Abelson, J. M., Sweetman, J., & Jackson, J. S. (2007). Prevalence and distribution of major depressive disorder in African Americans, Caribbean Blacks, and non-Hispanic Whites: Results from the National Survey of American Life. *Archives of General Psychiatry, 64*(3), 305–315.

World Health Organization. (2020, January 30). *Depression.* https://www.who.int/news-room/fact-sheets/detail/depression

Kara Beckett, DSW, LCSW, is a Licensed Clinical Social Worker and founder of the Georgia Center for Mental Wellness, LLC, in Atlanta, Georgia. She earned her Bachelor of Science degree in family studies from the University of Maryland, College Park; Master of Social Work degree from Howard University; and Doctor of Social Work degree from Rutgers University. She has more than 20 years of experience in the social work field. As Core Faculty at Walden University, Dr. Beckett advances the field by educating future social work professionals. Her areas of specialization include diversity, mood disorders, and trauma.

Chapter 10
Innovative Strategies to Engage Black Men in Research

Quienton L. Nichols

This chapter highlights the history of Black and Brown people and their experiences participating in government-funded activities with a laser focus view of Black men and their participation or lack thereof in research. Looking at such history provides a solid context from which to better understand the barriers that prevent Black men from participating in research studies. To understand and appreciate the innovative strategies to engage Black men in research, it is important to stress and outline barriers that affect their participation as well as the factors that influence the degree to which they participate in research studies. To better understand the history that marked the foundation of their involvement and created barriers affecting their participation, it helps to provide a full awareness of the strategies and techniques to engage Black men in research studies. This chapter concludes with key innovative strategies that those seeking to engage Black men in research can adopt as techniques to increase the participation of Black men in research studies.

Black Men in Research and Barriers to Engage in Research Studies

This section looks at Black men and their research participation and provides an understanding that explains their consternation and trepidation to participate in research. The underrepresentation of racial and ethnic groups in research is an existential crisis that has garnered the attention of many public and private key organizations. As such, the National Institutes of Health (NIH), Food and Drug Administration (FDA), Centers for Disease Control and Prevention (CDC), and the

Q. L. Nichols (✉)
School of Social Work, Fayetteville State University, Fayetteville, NC, USA
e-mail: qnichols@uncfsu.edu

© The Author(s), under exclusive license to Springer Nature Switzerland AG 2022
Y. D. Dyson et al. (eds.), *Black Men's Health*,
https://doi.org/10.1007/978-3-031-04994-1_10

Human Capital Initiative require the inclusion of women and minorities (Coker et al., 2009; Hagiwara et al., 2014). Although attitudes and behaviors regarding Black men's participation in research are often guided by misinformation about the details of the Tuskegee study, many Black men still do not participate in research studies and are reluctant to do so (Shavers et al., 2000; Freimuth et al., 2001).

The history of the use of African Americans as unwilling research subjects has been captured in the research literature (Diaz et al., 2008; Earl and Penney, 2001; Hagiwara et al., 2014; Rotimi et al., 2016) and in the hearts and minds of Black men as demonstrated by their reluctance to engage, participate, or involve themselves in research studies (Freimuth et al., 2001; Smith et al., 2007). The availability of Black men as compared to other racial and ethnic groups to recruit from communities of color for potential participation in research studies has drastically decreased. This decrease, in part, is due to the "missing man" phenomenon (Graham et al., 2018; Rotimi et al., 2016), which espouses that there are 83 Black men for every 100 Black women. Thereby equating that "17% of Black men are forcibly removed from their communities possibly due to factors such as mass incarceration and premature mortality" (Graham et al., 2018).

Research shows that people of color (Nápoles-Springer et al., 2000; Moorman et al., 1999) in general and Black men in particular (Byrd et al., 2011) have experienced a plethora of challenges preventing their participation in research studies. As a result, many factors, some of which include past experiences such as mistrust based on historical medical abuses, misrepresentation about the research participation (Shavers et al., 2001; Scharff et al., 2010); unethical behaviors (Barrett et al., 2017; Braunstein et al., 2008; Diaz et al., 2008), and fears such as the breach of confidentiality and not being told the truth about the research, are barriers or impediments to Black men participating in research (Byrd et al., 2011; Graham et al., 2018; Randolph et al., 2018).

In an article by Coker et al. (2009), extensive literature was conducted that involved African Americans' participation in research conducted in the medical field, nursing, mental health, and education from 1990 to 2007. Much of their research findings mirror reasons supporting why Black men fail to participate in some research studies. According to Barrett et al. (2017), barriers to recruitment and engaging in participation include the following:

(a) The effects of psychosocial, cultural, and economic factors as reasons for lower participation rates in research studies by African Americans.
(b) Fear and mistrust of research because of historical abuses in research and medical practice, such as the Tuskegee syphilis study is deeply entrenched in African American communities and remains a prominent reason that African Americans decide not to participate in research studies.
(c) Time and financial constraints.
(d) Discomfort with sharing personal information or having a stranger in one's home.
(e) Race of the recruiter.

(f) Family members serving as gatekeepers and discouraging participation.
(g) Lack of clinic and research team communication and engagement could be barriers to ensuring effective recruitment of African Americans in research (Barrett et al., 2017, p. 455).

Innovative and Best Practices to Engage Black Men in Research

The history of mistreatment of Black men in research is not as complicated as it is well documented (Earl & Penney, 2001; Diaz et al., 2008; Freimuth et al., 2001) and clearly outlined and communicates the distress that Black men endure in the name of scientific research. As much as those facts are true, it is also true that research is replete with well-documented strategies to engage minorities in the research process (Barrett et al., 2017; Fenton et al., 2009; Hagiwara et al., 2014), women (Smith et al., 2007), African Americans (Huang & Coker, 2010; Kerkorian et al., 2007), as well as Black men (Graham et al., 2018; Qualls, 2002; Randolph et al., 2018; Shavers et al., 2001). A great number of techniques, approaches and recommendations that are utilized to engage these groups are shared strategies (Braunstein et al., 2008; Barrett et al., 2017). In as much as this section highlights the strategies researchers and recruiters utilize to engage Black men in research (Barrett et al., 2017; Beatty et al., 2004; Kaplan et al., 2015; Graham et al., 2018), it also underscores the Men of Color Health Awareness (MOCHA) project's strategies in recruiting Black men in research (Graham et al., 2018). Identified as one of the Innovative Tailored-Recruitment Interventions (iTRI), this section also highlights and presents some of the Personalized Innovative Comprehensive (PIC) strategies to engage Black men in research.

Strategies that researchers adopt that address the fears, distrust, and concerns of Black men regarding confidentiality and privacy are worthwhile skill-building techniques to have in the toolbox. These toolbox techniques are identified as Intentional Tailored-research Techniques (ITT) and are grouped into two categories, which are personalized innovative comprehensive (PIC) and traditional innovative customary (TIC). Personalized innovative comprehensive (PIC) techniques are community-based specific, all-inclusive techniques that encourage the continuation of research participation. Traditional innovative customary (TIC) techniques are project-based specific techniques that identify recruitment barriers to research projects. It is important to note that intentional tailored-research techniques, personalized innovative comprehensive techniques, and the traditional innovative customary techniques are all strategies that are vital to recruiting and engaging Black men in research. Hence, the successful formula to recruiting and retaining Black men in research is iTRI + PIC + TIC = Success. Once adopted by researchers, this formula has the potential to address many barriers Black men face when participating in research, such as fears, distrust, issues with confidentiality, and concerns regarding privacy and are worthwhile skill-building techniques to have in the toolbox.

These toolbox strategies along with the techniques to encourage the continuation of research include the use of transparency, focused attention to time challenges and establishing rapport. Other strategies include adhering to cultural competency guidelines, practicing role-playing, and being up-front about historical atrocities affecting Black men. Lastly, adopting personalized recruitment strategies such as establishing longstanding personal ties, tabling at events and civic presence are actions that when taken can positively result in ways to engage Black men in research (Barrett et al., 2017; Graham et al., 2018; Byrd et al., 2011; Randolph et al., 2018).

Intentional Tailored-Research Techniques (ITT)

When working to engage Black men in research, it is essential to stress the importance of listening to the participants and not just hearing them. As researchers, the ability to identify resources to help support Black men and their families can be the result of listening and discerning their needs. As Barrett et al. (2017) puts it, "acknowledging the whole person" as an innovative strategy to engage African Americans in research and assisting Black men who decide to be participants in a research study with resources are also important and have the potential to result in them being more cooperative (Randolph et al., 2018; Barrett et al., 2017; Graham et al., 2018). An activity to support this strategy includes creating a community database of needed resources and making that database available to participants during the research and after it as well. Particularly if the plan is to solicit black male participants for future research.

Being mindful of participants' time is also crucial to recruitment and retention of Black men in research and adopting techniques to address concerns with time are needed strategies. Some of the strategies include modifying schedules to support time conflict issues and alter processes that would assist participants in seeing the research project to the end. This could include offering several different convenient locations to participate in the research or making alternate time opportunities to participate, such as on the weekends or during early morning or late evening hours (Barrett et al., 2017; Shavers et al., 2001; Randolph et al., 2018). Research shows that clinic personnel has a significant impact on the recruitment and retention of Black men in research (Byrd et al., 2011; Mason, 2005; Lang et al., 2013). For instance, if the research is of a medical nature, researchers should work to not only establish rapport but build rapport between the research team and key figures in the African American community. This serves as an important network to assist in recruiting patients and a vital strategy to employ.

Cultural competency and skillset building training as a strategy include incorporating cultural competency training to raise awareness around biases and cultural differences. Cultural diversity training to improve self-awareness of biases and strategies to think "outside-the-box" are excellent strategies to engage Black men in research. For example, in the MOCHA project, Black men who participated in the research reported receiving a "personal touch" in their participation in the research. Their responses were possibly a result of attention given to mirror the research facilitator's race, ethnicity, and communication style, which included familiar language, common vernacular and rhythm expressions (Graham et al., 2018). This practice of cultural congruence was highlighted as a strategy that encouraged Black men to participate in the research project (Randolph et al., 2018; Graham et al., 2018; Mason, 2005). Utilizing the practice of role-playing and other techniques to better the understanding of cultural issues by research team members demonstrates how to engage Black men participants in a mutually empowering way (Barrett et al., 2017).

Innovative Tailored-Recruitment Intervention (iTRI)

It is clearly documented that being of a different race or ethnicity than the study participant negatively affects the participation of minorities in research (Braunstein et al., 2008; Coker et al., 2009; Kaplan et al., 2015); challenges grow exponentially when recruiting and engaging Black men in research (Graham et al., 2018; Huang & Coker, 2010; Pariera et al., 2017). As a strategy, concerted efforts to include Black male researchers as team members when soliciting the support of Black male participants should be employed. Coined as the "For Me Like Me" strategy, this Innovative Tailored-Recruitment Intervention (iTRI) helps to overcome barriers of fear and mistrust because the research recruiters and the Black men asked to participate often times share the same race and ethnicity. Although simple but doable, this technique, along with adopting strategies, allows for more success in securing knowledge of skillsets and building rapport with the study participant. Additionally, because both the researcher and participants share the same race, finding a common point of interest is made just that easier.

To get more buy-in from Black men, research recruiters can express concerns about and be aware of issues Black men face regarding their distrust of medical research. Researchers should confront those issues and be upfront about the atrocities of the Tuskegee study and the grave harm it caused regarding Black men and their distrust in research (Shavers et al., 2001; Coker et al., 2009; Earl & Penney, 2001; Freimuth et al., 2001). Research recruiters should also demonstrate how their research team plans to build trusting relationships and ethically conduct research if given the opportunity to work with Black men (Shavers et al., 2001). Point of Understanding – The Tuskegee Study, symbolic of the larger problem of African American distrust of the white medical establishment, has evolved in the presence of racial discrimination, racial inequities in quality of care, and a previous history of medical research misuse (Shavers et al., 2000, p. 571).

The availability of Black men as compared to other racial and ethnic groups to recruit from other communities of color as potential participants in research studies has drastically decreased. The decrease, in part, is due to the "missing man" phenomenon (Graham et al., 2018). Point of Understanding – Innovative tailored-recruitment interventions (iTRI) are novel strategies utilized to recruit Black men for research participation. The purpose behind the need for Intentional Tailored-Research Techniques (ITT) is to engage Black men in research and gather data that would improve their lives and the lives of their families and their communities.

Personalized Innovative Comprehensive Strategies

Recruitment strategies that identify as Personalized – Innovative – Comprehensive (PIC) include personalized recruitment strategies that provide screenings at health fairs, work with community-based organizations as intermediaries, and conduct face-to-face recruitment, most commonly in churches. Others include face-to-face recruitment by ethnically matched staff conducting outreach in community-based organizations, with culturally tailored written correspondence and the use of barbershops to recruit Black men (Graham et al., 2018, p. 1309). Identified as an innovative tailored-recruitment intervention (iTRI) as well as an intentional tailored-research technique (ITT) for engaging Black men in research, the Men of Color Health Awareness (MOCHA) project is an excellent program to model and adopt.

Why the (MOCHA) Project?

Created to address issues that men of color face, enabling them to learn strategies to improve mental and emotional health and build social support networks with other men (Graham et al., 2018, p.1310), the Men of Color Health Awareness (MOCHA) project is an excellent program to model when engaging Black men in the research process. The MOCHA project is significant to the recruiting of Black men in research because of the innovative strategies it employs (Graham et al., 2018) and the benefits it can result in when engaging Black men in research (Barrett et al., 2017; Byrd et al., 2011; Graham et al., 2018; Hughes et al., 2017; Lang et al., 2013).

As one of the Innovative Tailored-Recruitment Intervention (iTRI) strategies, any research project with a goal to engage Black men in research can benefit from mirroring a model of action like the MOCHA project. Their outreach strategies are impressive and include:

> (a) tapping into existing social networks; (b) capitalizing on established relationships of trust; (c) appealing to join a broader movement for social change; and (d) enlisting past participants to become MOCHA mentors, thus setting off a snowball effect in expanding the reach of social networks, trust, and movement building (Graham et al., 2018, p. 1310).

The Men of Color Health Awareness (MOCHA) project goals are to:

(1) Reduce barriers to health care for men of color; (2) utilize the strengths inherent in cultural beliefs and norms regarding the role of men in caring for the health of their family; (3) enhance leadership among men of color in motivating change among their peers in behaviors that contribute to the onset of chronic diseases; (4) engage men of color in chronic disease self-management and wellness activities through peer-led activities; and (5) reduce poor health outcomes by building partnerships, implementing environmental strategies, and developing policies that create conditions for men of color to reach their full potential (Graham et al., 2018, p. 1310).

The outreach activities and social networks it adopts, such as tabling at events, its civic presence, and its "Brother Day celebration," are worth duplicating when working to recruit, engage and retain Black men in research (Graham et al., 2018).

The long-standing personal ties and connections enable MOCHA a head start in the arduous process of building trust, that most research projects face, and moving immediately into discussions about the benefits of participation (Graham et al., 2018, p. 1310). Its outreach is conducted by MOCHA mentors with well-established community ties. These men are oftentimes products of the community with wide-ranging social networks and bring extensive extended family ties in neighborhoods where the majority of the Black community lives (Graham et al., 2018, p. 1311). Tabling at events is where MOCHA mentors target events popular in the Black community, such as the Jazz Festival, the Stone Soul Picnic, and the Juneteenth Celebration. Juneteenth is a holiday celebrated on June 19 to commemorate the emancipation of enslaved people in the United States. The holiday was first celebrated in Texas, on that date in 1865 in the aftermath of the Civil War (Graham et al., 2018, p. 1312; Rotimi et al., 2016).

Civic presence is an innovative MOCHA strategy where time and resources are used to support causes and health promotion organizations in which they may not have a direct stake but will benefit the community in the long term (Graham et al., 2018, p. 1013). The recruiting methods by the MOCHA Project are innovative and worth underscoring, particularly when engaging the communities of Black men long term. Because of the clear and very doable steps with which to adopt them, researchers and recruiters can consider modeling the behaviors of MOCHA mentors (Graham et al., 2018). The MOCHA project is part of a larger movement, one that recognizes the need for social change, affecting change not only in the life of a Black man but also changing the social determinants of health of the Black man's community (Graham et al., 2018).

Summary

This chapter began by providing a cursory history of challenges and abuse faced by people of color and their participation in research with specific attention on Black men. It introduced barriers to engage in research studies and highlighted some as time concerns, discomfort with sharing personal information, the race of the recruiter, and lack of clinic and research team communication and engagement. It identified innovative best practices to engage Black men in research and provided techniques, approaches, and recommendation that research recruiters could utilize to engage Black men in research, some of which were categorized and grouped, which included intentional tailored-research techniques (ITT), personalized innovative comprehensive (PIC), and traditional innovative customary (TIC). The chapter concluded with a successful formula for recruiting and retaining Black men in research (iTRI + PIC + TIC = Success) and identified the Men of Color Health Awareness (MOCHA) project as an excellent program to model when engaging Black men in research studies.

Discussion Questions

1. In this chapter, strategies for researchers were addressed that could gain the trust and decrease some of the concerns of Black men in research. Identify and discuss these skill-building techniques, and explain how they can be utilized for the objective of increased participation of Black men in research.
2. Discuss the history of Black men and their experiences participating in research, and provide examples of Personalized Innovative Comprehensive (PIC) Strategies.
3. Discuss the impact that the MOCHA project has on the successful recruitment of Black men in research. Include in your response what the acronym means and at least three of the goals of the MOCHA project.

Exercises

The following exercises and activities invite students to review, explore further, and apply the methods discussed in the chapter. These activities can be done during or following the class, individually or in groups.

1. This chapter identified some examples of barriers Black men face in the participation of research. The Tuskegee study is an example of one of those barriers. The Tuskegee study is a historical reference for the mistrust of Black men in the participation of research. Explore and define what is the Tuskegee study and how the revelation of the study has an immediate impact on the Black community, especially Black men. Furthermore, identify other examples of medical research mistreatment of Black people that have impacted the mistrust of Black men to participate in the medical research community in your own communities.
2. In this chapter, strategies for researchers were addressed that could gain the trust and decrease some of the concerns of Black men in research. Identify these skill-building techniques and explain how they can be utilized for the objective of increased participation of Black men in research.
3. Brainstorm how you could work within your community, civic alliances, or personal relationships to engage, bring awareness, or foster positive attitudes in Black men for research participation. Some examples are mentioned in this chapter.
4. Discuss the two "Points of Understanding" located within the chapter content, and record a 60-s video of each and share it with your classmate. Be as creative and interesting as possible.

Glossary of Terms and Concepts

For Me Like Me: An Innovative Tailored-Recruitment Intervention (iTRI) strategy in which concerted efforts to include Black male researchers as team members when soliciting the support of Black men participants is utilized.

Innovative tailored-recruitment interventions (iTRI): Novel strategies utilized to recruit black men for research participation.

Intentional tailored-research techniques (ITT): Pioneering techniques utilized to encourage the continuation of participation in a research study.

Juneteenth: A holiday celebrated on June 19 to commemorate the emancipation of enslaved people in the United States. The holiday was first celebrated in Texas on that date in 1865 in the aftermath of the Civil War.

Missing man phenomenon: A trend that implies that Black men are forcibly removed from their communities possibly due to factors such as mass incarceration and premature mortality, thereby reducing the number of black men to participate in research studies.

Personalized innovative comprehensive (PIC): Community-based specific, all-inclusive techniques that encourage the continuation of research participation.

Traditional Innovative Customary (TIC): Project-based specific techniques that identify recruitment barriers to research.

References

Barrett, N. J., Ingraham, K. L., Vann Hawkins, T., & Moorman, P. G. (2017). Engaging African Americans in research: The recruiter's perspective. *Ethnicity & Disease, 27*(4), 453–462. https://doi-org.uncfsu.idm.oclc.org/10.18865/ed.27.4.453

Beatty, L. A., Wheeler, D., & Gaiter, J. (2004). HIV prevention research for African Americans: Current and future directions. *Journal of Black Psychology, 30*(1), 40–58. https://doi.org/10.1177/0095798403259245

Braunstein, J. B., Sherber, N. S., Schulman, S. P., Ding, E. L., & Powe, N. R. (2008). Race, medical researcher distrust, perceived harm, and willingness to participate in cardiovascular prevention trials. *Medicine, 87*(1), 1–9. https://doi.org/10.1097/MD.0b013e3181625d78

Byrd, G. S., Edwards, C. L., Kelkar, V. A., Phillips, R. G., Byrd, J. R., Pim-Pong, D. S., Starks, T. D., Taylor, A. L., Mckinley, R. E., Li, Y. J., & Pericak-Vance, M. (2011). Recruiting inter-generational African American males for biomedical research studies: A major research challenge. *Journal of the National Medical Association, 103*(6), 480–487. https://doi.org/10.1016/s0027-9684(15)30361-8

Coker, A. D., Huang, H.-H., & Kashubeck-West, S. (2009). Research with African Americans: Lessons learned about recruiting African American women. *Journal of Multicultural Counseling and Development, 37*(3), 153–165.

Diaz, V. A., Mainous, A. G., 3rd, McCall, A. A., & Geesey, M. E. (2008). Factors affecting research participation in African American college students. *Family Medicine, 40*(1), 46–51.

Earl, C. E., & Penney, P. J. (2001). The significance of trust in the research consent process with African Americans. *Western Journal of Nursing Research, 23*(7), 753–762. https://doi.org/10.1177/01939450122045528

Fenton, L., Rigney, M., & Herbst, R. S. (2009). Clinical trial awareness, attitudes, and participation among patients with cancer and oncologists. *Community Oncology, 6*(5), 207–228. https://doi.org/10.1016/S1548-5315(11)70546-0

Freimuth, V. S., Quinn, S. C., Thomas, S. B., Cole, G., Zook, E., & Duncan, T. (2001). African Americans' views on research and the Tuskegee Syphilis Study. *Social Science & Medicine (1982), 52*(5), 797–808. https://doi.org/10.1016/s0277-9536(00)00178-7

Graham, L. F., Scott, L., Lopeyok, E., Douglas, H., Gubrium, A., & Buchanan, D. (2018). Outreach strategies to recruit low-income African American men to participate in health promotion programs and research: Lessons from the men of color health awareness (MOCHA) project. *American Journal of Men's Health, 12*, 1307–1316. https://doi.org/10.1177/1557988318768602

Hagiwara, N., Berry-Bobovski, L., Francis, C., Ramsey, L., Chapman, R. A., & Albrecht, T. L. (2014). Unexpected findings in the exploration of African American underrepresentation in biospecimen collection and biobanks. *Journal of Cancer Education: The Official Journal of the American Association for Cancer Education, 29*(3), 580–587. https://doi.org/10.1007/s13187-013-0586-6

Huang, H., & Coker, A. D. (2010). Examining issues affecting African American participation in research studies. *Journal of Black Studies, 40*(4), 619–636. https://doi.org/10.1177/0021934708317749

Hughes, T. B., Varma, V., Pettigrew, C., & Albert, M. (2017). African Americans and clinical research: Evidence concerning barriers and facilitators to participation and recruitment recommendations. *The Gerontologist, 57*, 348–358.

Kaplan, C. P., Nápoles, A. M., Narine, S., Gregorich, S., Livaudais-Toman, J., Nguyen, T., Leykin, Y., Roach, M., & Small, E. J. (2015). Knowledge and attitudes regarding clinical trials and willingness to participate among prostate cancer patients. *Contemporary Clinical Trials, 45*(Pt B), 443–448. https://doi.org/10.1016/j.cct.2015.09.023

Kerkorian, D., Traube, D. E., & McKay, M. M. (2007). Understanding the African American Research Experience (KAARE): Implications for HIV Prevention. *Social Work in Mental Health, 5*(3 & 4), 295–312. https://doi.org/10.1300/J200v05n03_03

Lang, R., Kelkar, V. A., Byrd, J. R., Edwards, C. L., Pericak-Vance, M., & Byrd, G. S. (2013). African American participation in health-related research studies: Indicators for effective recruitment. *Journal of Public Health Management and Practice : JPHMP, 19*(2), 110–118. https://doi.org/10.1097/PHH.0b013e31825717e

Mason, S. E. (2005). Offering African Americans opportunities to participate in clinical trials research: How social workers can help. *Health & Social Work, 30*, 296–304.

Moorman, P. G., Newman, B., Millikan, R. C., Tse, C. K., & Sandler, D. P. (1999). Participation rates in a case-control study: The impact of age, race, and race of interviewer. *Annals of Epidemiology, 9*(3), 188–195. https://doi.org/10.1016/s1047-2797(98)00057-x

Nápoles-Springer, A. M., Grumbach, K., Alexander, M., Moreno-John, G., Forté, D., Rangel-Lugo, M., & Pérez-Stable, E. J. (2000). Clinical research with older African Americans and Latinos: Perspectives from the community. *Research on Aging, 22*(6), 668–691. https://doi.org/10.1177/0164027500226004

Pariera, K. L., Murphy, S. T., Meng, J., & McLaughlin, M. L. (2017). Exploring willingness to participate in clinical trials by ethnicity. *Journal of Racial and Ethnic Health Disparities, 4*(4), 763–769. https://doi.org/10.1007/s40615-016-0280-6

Qualls, C. D. (2002). Recruitment of African American adults as research participants for a language in aging study: Example of a principled, creative, and culture-based approach. *Journal of Allied Health, 31*(4), 241–246.

Randolph, S., Coakley, T., & Shears, J. (2018). Recruiting and engaging African American men in health research. *Nurse Researcher, 26*(1), 8–12. https://doi.org/10.7748/nr.2018.e1569

Rotimi, C. N., Tekola-Ayele, F., Baker, J. L., & Shriner, D. (2016). The African diaspora: History, adaptation and health. *Current opinion in genetics & development, 41*, 77–84. https://doi.org/10.1016/j.gde.2016.08.005

Scharff, D. P., Mathews, K. J., Jackson, P., Hoffsuemmer, J., Martin, E., & Edwards, D. (2010). More than Tuskegee: Understanding mistrust about research participation. *Journal of Health Care for the Poor and Underserved, 21*(3), 879–897. https://doi.org/10.1353/hpu.0.0323

Shavers, V. L., Lynch, C. F., & Burmeister, L. F. (2000). Knowledge of the Tuskegee study and its impact on the willingness to participate in medical research studies. *Journal of the National Medical Association, 92*(12), 563–572.

Shavers, V. L., Lynch, C. F., & Burmeister, L. F. (2001). Factors that influence African-Americans' willingness to participate in medical research studies. *Cancer, 91*(1 Suppl), 233–236. https://doi.org/10.1002/1097-0142(20010101)91:1+<233::aid-cncr10>3.0.co;2-8

Smith, Y. R., Johnson, A. M., Newman, L. A., Greene, A., Johnson, T. R., & Rogers, J. L. (2007). Perceptions of clinical research participation among African American women. *Journal of Women's Health (2002), 16*(3), 423–428. https://doi.org/10.1089/jwh.2006.0124

Quienton L. Nichols, PhD, is the Associate Dean and Associate Professor of Social Work in the School of Social Work at Fayetteville State University (FSU) in North Carolina. He received his Bachelor and Master of Social Work degrees from the University of Georgia, School of Social Work, in Athens, Georgia, and his PhD in Social Work Administration, Planning and Social Science from Clark Atlanta University, Whitney M. Young School of Social Work, in Atlanta, Georgia. Dr. Nichols's academic administration includes MSW Director at FSU, Director of the Child Welfare Scholars Program, and Director of Field Education at Kennesaw State University in Kennesaw, Georgia.

Part IV
Social Justice Implications for Black Men's Health

Chapter 11
Social Justice and Black Men's Health

Shonda K. Lawrence, Jerry Watson, Kristie Lipford, Nathaniel Currie, and Malik Cooper

A 3-year drop in life expectancy for all Black Americans during the pandemic in 2020 created a 6-year gap between Black and White Americans (Pullano, 2021). However, negative health outcomes for Black men are even more alarming and concerning. Studies have found lack men mortality risk for stroke is 70% greater than white men (Summary Health Statistics [CDC], 2021); they have the shortest life expectancy of all race/gender groups (National Center for Health Statistics, 2019); and they die younger than all other groups of men, except for Native Americans, (Gadson, 2006; Warner, 2006). The painful and disturbing fact is that Black men have the worst health outcomes when compared to other racial/ ethnic groups in the United States. Lung cancer is the second most common cancer in Black men, and they are more than twice as likely to die from prostate cancer than White men (American Cancer Society, 2019–2021; Stuart, 2019). Black men are also nine times more likely to die from AIDS than their White counterparts (Gilbert et al., 2016); and among young Black men, the mortality rate for homicides is 51.5 per 100,000 of the population compared with 2.9 per 100,000 of the population for their White counterparts (Center for Disease Control and Prevention, 2019). On the topics of diagnoses, health management, and health-seeking behavior, Black men are more likely than other racial and ethnic groups to have undiagnosed or poorly managed chronic conditions (cancer, diabetes, hypertension, heart disease) and more

S. K. Lawrence (✉) · N. Currie · M. Cooper
Whitney M. Young Jr. School of Social Work, Clark Atlanta University, Atlanta, GA, USA
e-mail: slawrence@cau.edu; ncurrie@cau.edu; malik.cooper@students.cau.edu

J. Watson
School of Social Work, University of Memphis, Memphis, TN, USA
e-mail: jerry.watson@memphis.edu

K. Lipford
Urban Studies & Health Equity Programs, Rhodes College, Memphis, TN, USA
e-mail: lipfordk@rhodes.edu

© The Author(s), under exclusive license to Springer Nature Switzerland AG 2022
Y. D. Dyson et al. (eds.), *Black Men's Health*,
https://doi.org/10.1007/978-3-031-04994-1_11

likely to delay seeking medical treatment (Griffith et al., 2013; Jackson & Knight, 2006; Warner & Hayward, 2006; Williams, 2003). Black men's poor health outcomes, particularly when compared to their white counterparts, is critically important because men's health is important.

Current literature highlights seven prevailing social determinants that black men face when interacting with American healthcare systems. These seven social determinants include: (1) the *racism and mistrust* that is inherent within the medical industry; (2) the role *finances and economic stability* play in achieving health and wellness; (3) the desire to maintain and uphold *gender-influenced stereotypes*; (4) the influence *religion/faith-based ideologies* have on health and wellness; (5) the *lack of awareness* Black men have around managing their personal health; (6) the impact of *incarceration;* and (7) *Black male representation in medicine*. Altogether, these factors create a maze of issues Black men are expected to navigate and a mountain of challenges they must overcome when striving to obtain health and wellness.

The social and political enactments "against black Americans are enduring versions of institutional forces that manufacture and maintain health disparities" (Gilbert et al., 2016). The negative impact of social determinants on health equity for Black men is not a phenomenon leading one to question how or why. Rather, it is a condition of sociopolitical influences' subsequent impact on the state of Black men's health today. The central themes that course through the historical events related to healthcare and Black men are mistreatment, devaluation, and stark evidence of disparity. From slavery to the present day, the Black man has borne unspeakable applications of destruction to body and soul. It is important to understand and be knowledgeable of Black men's lived experiences along with the role that institutions within our ecosystem have played and the complexities of those interactions. In this chapter, social determinants, critical race theory (CRT), and intersectionality theory provide a solid basis for conceptualization and understanding of this dilemma.

Racism and Mistrust

While racist systems and practices are commonplace in American institutions, it is especially pervasive and intrusive within the field of medicine. Healthcare systems, that once used Black men as subjects of scientific experimentation, have embedded a manifestation of negative and harmful interactions that make it difficult for Black men to establish a trusting relationship with the healthcare system. The prevalence of racism and mistrust of the healthcare system has had a profound impact on health outcomes for Black men. Countless studies have pointed to racism and mistrust of the medical industry as primary factors that significantly influence Black men's overall health and wellness (Brandt, 1978; Fowler-Brown et al., 2006). In Armstrong et al. (2007), a study examining racial/ethnic differences in physician distrust, Black men consistently reported higher mean levels of distrust of physicians than Whites.

A recent study titled *Medical Mistrust, Racism, and Delays in Preventive Health Screening Among African American Men* found that the mistrust of healthcare providers, coupled with the personal and painful experiences of racism, makes Black men more likely to put off health screenings and routine doctor's appointments (Powell et al., 2019). Similar studies consistently found that Black people are more likely than White people to admit that they were fearful of being experimented on while in the hospital, more likely to believe that a study like that of the Tuskegee experiment could happen again, and less likely than their White counterparts to trust their physicians and other medical professionals (Fowler-Brown et al., 2006; Watson, 2014; Boulware et al., 2003; Blocker et al., 2006). Whether real or perceived, racial biases/racism contribute to the mistrust Black men have of the medical system. As a result, black men are choosing not to seek preventative healthcare (Powell et al., 2019), and significant numbers of Black men may not be getting the medical care and treatment needed to maintain healthy lives.

Finances and Economic Stability

Black men have the highest unemployment rates of any race/gender group (Holzer, 2021), and unemployment is associated with higher levels of stress and illness (Pharr et al., 2012). Employment continues to be an issue for people who are positioned at the lower end of the socioeconomic scale. Socioeconomic status (personal finances, income, and inability to afford healthcare services) is consistently cited in the literature as a significant barrier Black man face when attempting to achieve optimal health and wellness (Royster et al., 2006; Serota et al., 2019; Whitaker et al., 2018; Ravenell et al., 2008). Aside from urgent medical care, Black men who experience financial issues may endure a host of unmet and unresolved medical concerns because of their inability to afford treatment and having to weigh loss of wages and medical treatment.

Gender-Influenced Stereotypes

Gender-influenced stereotypes, particularly those associated with the male gender identity, are cited as another major barrier that influences the health outcomes of Black men. Gender identity is loosely defined as a person's conception of oneself as cisgender male or female, transgender male or female, or outside the gender binary, also known as gender nonbinary. Gender identity is intimately related to the concept of gender role, which is defined as the outward manifestations of personality that reflect the gender identity. For Black men, in today's America, gender identity is associated with virility, masculinity, physical and emotional strength, risk-taking, toughness, boldness, and bravery. The intentional preservation of these stereotypes explains why medical service utilization among Black men is low. The Powell,

Adams, Cole-Lewis, Agyemang, and Upton study (2016) further affirms this by noting that gender-influenced stereotypes, like those mentioned above, have a profound impact on men's identities and their help-seeking behaviors. Their article titled *Masculinity and Race-Related Factors as Barriers to Health Help-Seeking Among African American Men*, Powell et al. explains that "as a multidimensional set of social prescriptions, masculinity norms theoretically encourage men to avoid help-seeking, display emotional stoicism or toughness, cope autonomously, and maintain a high sense of control even in the face of negative life experiences" (p. 151). Their study essentially found that the reason for help-seeking avoidance is that events, symptoms, or external cues signaling healthcare need threaten masculine identity, diminish sense of control, and increase men's need to engage in behavior designed to restore freedom (Powell et al., 2016). And so, for many Black men, the act of seeking healthcare can be seen as a weak and undesirable character trait. Fear of embarrassment, invasion of privacy, invasion of bodies, and fear of assault on their manhood are all noted as barriers that explain healthcare disparities (Blocker et al., 2006).

Religion/Faith-Based Ideology

Religious influence and general spiritual beliefs have emerged in the literature as factors that potentially impact health disparities among African American men. Religion and faith-based ideology emerged in the literature as both an obstacle to and an encourager of Black men's health-seeking behaviors. One study found that for some believers, their body is God's temple. These believers, therefore, feel obligated to care for themselves and their bodies. In cases like this, health maintenance is seen to be in alignment with God's will and His plan for one's life. These individuals were more likely to schedule doctor appointments and properly follow healthcare plans (Blocker et al., 2006). In instances where faith-based theology is seen as an obstacle to healthcare, black men believers were less likely to schedule doctor appointments and less likely to comply with doctor's orders because they either have accepted illness as part of God's plan or they understand illness to be a punishment for bad deeds. Those with this belief system were less likely to take medications and engage in health-seeking behaviors as well (Rose et al., 2000).

Positive benefits of religion due to its buffering effects and the positive coping mechanisms it provides are significant for African American health because African Americans tend to report higher religious involvement and affiliation than other racial groups. Furthermore, research has also shown that African Americans use religion to cope with health issues. From an institutional perspective, the Black Christian Church has remained a consistent fixture in African American life. Past studies have examined the role of the Black Church in supporting African American men's health (Allen et al., 2010; Rowland & Isaac-Savage, 2014; Collins & Perry, 2015). Robinson et al., (2018) provides a balanced, yet critical perspective on the involvement of the church in men's health. The authors suggest that Black churches expand their involvement to include discussions on social stressors and justice issues (Robinson et al., 2018).

Personal Health Management

A qualitative study (2008) identifying barriers to health care among Black men reported lack of awareness as a barrier to Black men engaging in health-seeking behaviors for disease signs and symptoms. The focus group participant shared, "disease related to our nationality, to our race, you don't see the symptoms...some of the things that come to my mind is hypertension and prostate problems and now something else that is coming up quite regular is colon cancer. What is the prevention for that? What are the signs? What are the early symptoms of it?" (Ravenell et al., 2008, p. 1155).

If this information is unknown, then Black men may not be properly positioned to seek care for themselves and others. Another study found that Black men only sought medical care when the condition inhibited their normal and daily functioning. The men were known to delay treatment until their condition worsened; and many of them opted to use emergency care treatment at the last minute instead of deciding to use preventative care methods (Blocker et al., 2006; Forrester-Anderson, 2005; Plowden & Young, 2003; Whetten et al., 2006). The failure to seek medical care speaks to the general lack of knowledge and health awareness that exists among this population. Awareness of personal health and well-being is key and serves as an integral part of becoming healthy.

Incarceration

Slavery showed the brutal and cruel physical treatment of Black people in this country that propagated the belief that Black people were inferior, not human, and were to be treated as such. The propagation of this belief continued after slavery with the codification of racist laws during the Jim Crow era in southern states, lynching, and de facto segregation. Although the Civil Rights Act of 1964 prohibits healthcare systems receiving federal financing and support from employing discriminatory practices based on race or color, discrimination in the American healthcare system is evidence of the poor implementation of the law to date (Frakt, 2020). These social and political acts have set the tone for how Black men are perceived and treated in the health care system today.

An example is the political response to drug use/abuse, known as the Anti-Drug Abuse Act of 1986 or "War on Drugs," and its devastating impact on black communities. Although Black communities are not more likely to use or sell drugs than any other community, Blacks are more likely to be arrested and incarcerated for drug offenses. We are still experiencing the impact of the Act as expansion of the prison industrial complex garnered a significant increase in the number of incarcerated Black men. Further, Black men are six times more likely than White men to be incarcerated (National Urban League, 2007). With the recent COVID-19 pandemic looming and inadequate provisions of health care in prison settings, incarceration has amplified health inequity for black men. So, while incarceration can be seen as a separate factor impacting Black men's health outcomes, "racial disparities in our criminal justice system flow directly into economic inequality" (Craigie et al., 2020, p. 6) and disparity in health provisions.

Black Male Representation in Medicine

Increasing medical representation is one solution to improving Black men's health. Only 3% of medical providers are Black men (AAMC, 2015), even though Black men have some of the highest rates of diseases (Arias et al., 2018). Laurencin and Murray (2017) refer to the lack of diversity among medical providers as an American crisis. An obvious contributor to low Black male representation is the reduced number of Black male applicants to medical school since the start of the twenty-first century (AAMC, 2015). Only half of those who apply enroll in medical school (AAMC, 2015), and the numbers are even lower for US-born Black males. This is indeed an American crisis because limited diversity in health care decreases quality of care for all patients (Laurencin and Murray, 2017; Walker et al., 2012). Most African American physicians enter primary care specialties. However, the literature and national data on racial representation in medical specialties are scant (Rotenstein et al., 2021). One study does manage to explore associations between race, specialty, and likelihood of working in an underserved area. These researchers found that Black and Latino doctors, compared to Whites, are more likely to work in underserved areas. Also, nearly half of Black doctors worked in primary care (Walker et al., 2007).

Surgery is vastly underrepresented with roughly 6% as general surgery residents (Abelson et al., 2018). One study conducted by University of Pennsylvania researchers explored the barriers that medical students face when selecting academic surgery as a specialty (Roberts et al., 2020). The researchers interviewed 16 African American men and women. Findings revealed that common barriers were financial responsibilities, being employed in predominantly White workplaces, stress, limited mentorship, insecurity, and feeling undervalued. The researchers concluded that low African American representation in academic surgery is multifactorial and requires an array of solutions to reduce barriers for Black doctors who desire to enter the surgical field.

Academic psychiatry also has very limited diversity. In 2015, only 141 of the psychiatry faculty identified as African American (AAMC, 2017; Taylor et al., 2009). This is also another specialty where providers do not adequately reflect the racial make-up of the communities most in need. The low representation is extremely important when mental health issues among Black men are considered. Population data show Black men have high rates of anxiety and depression (Smith et al., 2011). Data also suggests that mental distress is higher in younger Black men (Lincoln et al., 2011; Sellers et al., 2009). Black male suicide is also increasing in the United States (Chatters et al., 2011). Despite the high rates of mental health conditions, Black men are less likely to access mental health resources. Because mental health crises are increasing and the practicing number of Black men in the field remains low, there have been calls to establish community-based interventions to address Black male mental health (Watkins et al., 2017). Another key specialty where Black men suffer disparities or make up a disproportionate share of patient populations is prostate cancer. Racial gaps are observed in prostate cancer incidence, severity, and mortality (Jindal et al., 2017; Mahal et al., 2017), yet only 2% of practicing urologists are Black (Vince et al., 2020). Research suggests that Black men with Black doctors are more likely to be screened due to greater trust and communication. One study found that Black men with Black doctors had more invasive screenings and engaged in more preventive care services (Alsan et al., 2019).

There are many contributing factors that impact low Black male representation in medicine. One issue with low representation of Black men in medicine is the missed opportunities to mentor. Mentorship in medicine is associated with several positive career outcomes. Medical trainees and doctors who have mentors are more likely to receive promotions, engage in research, and report more career satisfaction (Bhatnagar et al., 2020; Jackson & Knight, 2006). Other research has shown the importance of minority mentors and social support as significant contributors to Black male success in medical school (Thomas et al., 2019; Thurmond & Cregler, 1999). Another contributing factor is financial challenges. Recent AMA (2015) data suggests that 75% of medical graduates have debt incurred from medical school. Financial concerns were cited as a major obstacle for a large majority of a student sample (Rao & Flores, 2007). Specifically, students listed the high cost of tuition. In addition, students negatively perceived the debt they incur and attainment of academic scholarship as a challenging feat. African American students also perceived scholarship contributions as limited (Rao & Flores, 2007) and that financial roadblocks are the biggest barriers that racial minorities face in applying to medical schools (Hadinger, 2017). Finally, minority students consistently report microaggressions (Chisholm et al., 2020). Microaggressions are subtle and hidden racial messaging and behaviors that occur in interpersonal interactions (Almond, 2019). One study found that medical students perceive racial microaggressions as a part of their daily school and clinical experiences. Students also reported that these experiences cause great mental distress (Ackerman-Barger et al., 2020). Racial microaggressions also negatively influence clinical learning settings, and students who experience these microaggressions often have lower academic performance and engagement (Ackerman-Barger et al., 2020; Chisholm et al., 2020).

Critical Race Theory Overview

In the late 1970s, several forward-thinking American lawyers, activists, and legal scholars recognized that they needed a new framework to combat racism and oppression in America. These early scholars, like Derrick Bell, Kimberlé Crenshaw,

Richard Delgado, and Alan Freeman (among others), blended concepts from critical legal studies and radical feminism with the influences of the Black Power and Chicano movements of the time to create a framework and lens known as *critical race theory*. Early critical race theory (CRT), also known as critical race studies (CRS), was mainly referenced in legal scholarship, but today it is used across many different fields and disciplines, including academia, social work and other helping professions, and social policy, having become an academic movement in the 1980s, and having seen a mainstream interest in the early 2000s. Critical race theory asks us to consider how we can transform the relationship between race, racism, and power and work toward the liberation of BIPOC (Black, Indigenous, People of Color) communities. CRT also seeks to challenge mainstream liberal approaches to social justice work. We will explore this further in the five tenets that make up the CRT framework.

Although the original focus was on the African American/Black experience of race and racism which is normalized and enmeshed in the fabric of American social order (Ladson-Billings, 1998). CRT has since been applied internationally across diverse social contexts where people are minoritized due to race, gender, class, sexual orientation, or other "axes of differentiation" (Gillborn & Ladson-Billings, 2010). CRT is not only interested in overt manifestations of oppression but in the nuanced and hidden mechanisms of power and its maintenance that disadvantage some groups while privileging others (Gillborn, 2006). CRT seeks to unearth and hold accountable the profound patterns of exclusion that exist in US society. It is no wonder that CRT has gained such popularity in the helping professions; the framework itself parallels many of the values, ethics, and calls to action of social work practice, medicine, and sociology.

Critical race theory (CRT) is regularly conceptualized as five main tenets that create a lens for which to examine. The five tenets of CRT include: (1) the social construction of race; (2) the notion that racism is permanent in American culture, it is ordinary and not aberrational; (3) interest convergence; (4) storytelling and counter-storytelling; and (5) the critique of liberalism. Some scholars include/ exclude: (A) Whiteness as property and (B) the social construct of race. To organize this theory for the helping professions, we will discuss Whiteness as property under the critique of liberalism. Let us look at the major components of each tenet.

The social construct of race is best described first as understanding that a social construct is something that exists not in objective reality, but because of human interaction. It exists because humans agree that it exists. Scientists have found that there is no mitochondrial DNA explanation for race, therefore suggesting that race, as it were, is socially constructed. In American society, the acceptance and use of race have clear economic, power, class, and cultural benefits for some while excluding others. CRT examines these concepts fully and acknowledges their importance in American society, particularly in how they exclude or oppress vulnerable communities.

Racism is permanent or racism is ordinary, not aberrational, as in the usual way US society has structured economy, power, and culture, as well as the common, everyday experience of most people of color in this country is embedded with racist ideology and often behavior. Further, White supremacy creates both a material and psychological hierarchy, also embedded into US society and culture. Ordinary formal conceptions of equality expressed in rules made through policy and law can only remedy the most blatant forms of discrimination, leaving the more salient and widely practiced, sometimes unacknowledged forms unaddressed. CRT seeks to alleviate this structure(s) as work toward liberation.

Interest convergence is the notion that Whites will support racial justice/progress to the extent that there is something positive in it for them, or a "convergence" between the interests of Whites and non-White/BIPOC and/or non-cisgender hetero-identified communities. Interests may include power, control, economy, and use, hoarding, or access to resources.

Storytelling and counter-storytelling the idea of storytelling comes from its powerful, persuasive, and explanatory ability to unlearn beliefs that are commonly believed to be true. Counter-storytelling is a method of telling a story that aims to cast doubt on the validity of accepted premises or myths, especially ones held by the majority. Think about who writes the history books and controls mass media, what perspective do they hold? How does their storytelling benefit their histories and trajectories?

Counter-storytelling is a tool that CRT scholars employ to contradict racist characterizations of social life and expose race-neutral discourse, revealing how White privilege operates to reinforce and support unequal racial relations in society. While majoritarian stories draw on the tacit knowledge among persons in the dominant group (Delgado et al., 2017), they also distort and silence the experiences of the dominated. What other dominant narratives/ideologies exist that contribute to intersectional oppression? Think about this as you read through the intersectional theory of this chapter.

Critique of liberalism stems from critique of basic notions embraced by liberal legal ideology to include colorblindness and meritocracy (a mechanism that allows people to ignore racist policies that perpetuate social inequity) and neutrality of law (that racism is codified in law, embedded in systems and political structure, and to ignore race does not show neutrality). Color-blindness and meritocratic rhetoric serve two primary functions; first, they allow Whites to feel consciously irresponsible for the hardships BIPOC communities face and encounter daily; and second, they also maintain Whites' power and strongholds within society. Think about how these concepts are important to the holding of power and resources.

Whiteness as property, sometimes considered a core CRT tenet, looks at the history of race and racism in the United States and the role US jurisprudence has played in reifying concepts of race; the notion of Whiteness can be considered a property interest (Harris, 1993). This concept furthers the notion that Whites have actually been recipients of civil rights legislation, even as theprimary beneficiaries of civil rights legislation. Take for instance Affirmative Action (Executive Order No. 10925, signed by President John F. Kennedy, March 6, 1961)—who has most benefited from this policy and why? Does gender play a role in this examination? Why or why not?

Intersectional theory, or intersectionality, as it is commonly referred, is the examination of race, sex, gender, class, national origin, and sexual orientation and how their combination or their intersection plays out in various settings. Further, this concept identifies that no person has a single, easily stated, unitary identity, but that intersectionality and anti-essentialism are ever present, whereas everyone has overlapping, conflicting identities and loyalties. Intersectionality theory also highlights an emphasis on individuals' experiences and within-group differences.

CRT Application: African American Men and American Healthcare Experience

African American/Black men have a unique and often painful history with the US healthcare system, as with virtually all care and support systems, as you will see as we explore the topic more diversely and in depth throughout this chapter. Likewise, we could choose to look at any health issue or disparity through a critical race lens and find similar outcomes for African American/Black men. HIV (human immunodeficiency virus) is a good example for practicing both the use of the CRT lens as well as the necessity for it. Centers for Disease Control and Prevention data state that African Americans/Blacks make up 13% of the total US population but represent 42% of new (2018) HIV diagnoses. This number is held predominantly by African American/Black men with 11,900 new HIV acquisitions in comparison to just over 4000 new HIV acquisitions for African American/Black women for the same year (2018).

The socioeconomic issues associated with poverty—including limited access to high-quality health care and educated use of health care and health insurance systems, stable affordable housing, and HIV prevention education and prevention resources (including biomedical prevention interventions, like pre- and post-exposure prophylaxis, also known as PrEP and PEP)—directly and indirectly increase the risk for HIV infection and affect the overall health of African American/Black men living with HIV. These factors may explain why BIPOC communities and, in particular, African American/Black men have worse outcomes on the HIV continuum of care, including lower rates of linkage to care, use of mental health systems, and viral suppression, a key measure in health, wellness, and long-term survival of HIV/AIDS.

Critical race theory pushes professionals in the helping professions to question data, systems, leadership within systems, care, and education access and requires practitioners to identify and possibly address instances where marginal communities are not included in solutions at all system levels. CRT lens-based examination suggests that African American/Black men, community members, and leaders alike must be included in HIV prevention, education, and care efforts. Leaders of organizations representing marginal communities are allowed on occasion, conditional entrance and limited power in dominant institutions and decision-making. This allowance comes with the unspoken understanding that these leaders represent the views and temper the actions of the marginal group (Cohen, 1999). Efforts to address provisional and/or radical entrance into system decision-making spaces, and healthcare engagement, are furthered through a CRT framework.

Summary

This chapter provides a brief overview of the literature emphasizing the seven unique and prevailing obstacles and barriers that Black men face when interacting with healthcare systems. Issues of racism and mistrust, finances and economic stability, gender-influenced stereotypes, religion/faith-based ideology, personal health management, incarceration, and Black men representation in medicine are believed to be the seven factors that provide an explanation for why Black men continue to experience poor health outcomes. The chapter discusses social and political factors that have had implications for how Black men interact with healthcare systems and utilizes the integrated lenses of critical race theory and intersectionality theory to conceptualize processes for understanding and change. Discussion questions and case studies are included to prompt critical thinking and elicit discussions on historical and structural racism, the influence of sociopolitical systems, and the implications for social work policy and practice.

Discussion Questions

1. When were you first aware of yourself as a member of _____ group? When were you first aware of people from other groups in this category? When did you first experience being treated differently because of your membership in this group? What did these experiences teach you about race/ethnicity/identity?
2. Can you think of a time when you struggled or were denied access to healthcare or medical treatment? What were some of the precipitating factors that lead to those experiences?
3. Can you identify a personal or public health issue that has been politicized? How did race show up in that issue?
4. Use the internet to search for three medical school mission or value statements. Critically evaluate the statements. What efforts do the statements convey? Do they include efforts to increase diversity in medicine?

Exercises

When addressing structural and systemic racism with advocacy efforts for policy changes at the state and federal levels, it is important that persons working in the healthcare field are knowledgeable and acknowledge, in practice, the experiences of Black men. A strengths-based approach that includes active listening, comfortability, use of language, patient participation, responsiveness, follow-up, and advocacy are skills that support the provision of adequate health care and engagement with Black men. Review the engagement framework provided for you in Table 11.1. Read the case studies (Case Studies 11.1 and 11.2).[1]

---

[1] To protect privacy/confidentiality, all names and other personal identifiers in the case studies are fictitious and do not represent any real person or situation.

Using the engagement framework, critical race theory, and intersectional theory, identify the issues, assess, and discuss what interventions could facilitate a different outcome. Provide a rationale for your answer.

Case Study 11.1

Mr. Calhoun, a 46-year-old Black man, has presented in the emergency room with sharp stomach pains and a temperature of 102 and reports of "spitting up blood." He has been suffering from stomach pains for approximately 1 month. He reports that he has not seen a doctor since he was 17 years old. During his childhood, he had only visited a doctor's office for a yearly physical as required by the school. He is very nervous and does not trust doctors or the healthcare system. He is a religious man and believes that prayer can heal. He only decided to come to the emergency room at the urgency of his wife.

Mr. Calhoun reports that he has a family history of men suffering from stomach issues on the paternal side of his family. Although his father suffered from stomach issues, he believes the issues were controlled with over-the-counter medications. His father was diagnosed as having cancer at the age of 49. He was not sure what

Table 11.1 Engagement framework

Knowledge	Healthcare provider is knowledgeable about outcomes of medications, research, medical trials, etc. for black men. Healthcare provider is knowledgeable of the inclusion of the representative number of black maletrial/research/study participants.
Listening	Healthcare provider establishes an environment where the patient believes that the provider is listening and considering their healthcare concerns and needs. Eye contact and self-determination are very important.
Comfortability	Healthcare provider builds a rapport with the patient to facilitate a level of comfort for sharing personal, embarrassing, historical information related to healthcare needs. Nonverbal communication is very important.
Language	Healthcare provider uses language that can be understood and clearly explained for prognosis, diagnosis, and treatment.
Patient participation	Healthcare provider sustains a participatory environment where the patient actively participates in course of action for addressing healthcare needs. Healthcare provider is aware and implements processes for informed consent.
Responsiveness	Healthcare provider answers patients' questions and concerns in a reasonable period. The reasonable period should be no more than 48 h. However, if the response time is longer than 48 h, it is up to the healthcare provider to inform the patient of a normal response time at the first point of contact. Healthcare provider is aware of patient limitations related to using computer technology and their ability to accessphone and computer application communications.
Follow-up	Healthcare provider contacts patients after recommendation of treatment, during treatment, and conclusion of treatment to discuss patients' healthcare concerns and needs.
Advocacy	Healthcare provider is knowledgeable of past, present, and future healthcare policies that specifically impact healthcare provisions for Black men. Healthcare providers are actively engaged in advocating for equity and fairness in the development, lobbying, and implementation of healthcare policies

type of cancer caused his father's death. Mr. Calhoun's father refused treatment and later died at home when he was just a boy. His grandfather died at the age of 39. He reports that his grandfather went to the doctor for a routine physical for new employment. During the physical, his grandfather reported that he sometimes had issues with his stomach but controlled it by adjusting his dietary intake of spicy foods. The doctors enrolled him in an experimental medical trial to treat ulcers. According to Mr. Calhoun, his grandfather was not informed that the medication he was receiving was experimental. He died 1 month later of a heart attack. The family has always believed that it was the experimental medication that caused his death. Mr. Calhoun does not know the frequency at which his grandfather used doctors or medical facilities but reports that he can never remember his father going to the doctor except for the time he was diagnosed with cancer.

Mr. Calhoun has a wife and four children. He lives in a moderate home, works for a small trucking company, and has medical insurance. His wife drove him to the emergency room and was present for intake of the patient. Mr. Calhoun's emergency room doctor does not have time to read Mr. Calhoun's background. The doctor gives him a brief examination and treats his symptoms. Mr. Calhoun is given a white substance to drink. The doctor instructs the nurse to give Mr. Calhoun a referral for a follow-up appointment, asks that he set up an online medical profile so that he can access his medical and billing records and referral information. He is stabilized and refused further treatment. He states that he does not trust the doctor because he never looked at him or asked him any questions. Mr. and Mrs. Calhoun leave the facility. Mr. Calhoun decides that he will not follow up with the referral and tells his wife to "just leave me alone about it."

Case Study 11.2

Read the case study. Identify the issues, assess, and discuss. What is your role as a practitioner? What barriers might you encounter? How did you use critical race theory and intersectionality in your thought process?

Mr. Jones, a 52-year-old Black man, has been diagnosed with end-stage kidney disease. His treatment plan includes dietary restrictions and receiving hemodialysis, a procedure that artificially removes waste products and extra fluid from the blood when the kidneys can no longer do this. Mr. Jones is scheduled for dialysis treatment three times a week, 3–5 h per day. Mr. Jones is employed; however, his employer does not provide health insurance coverage. Mr. Jones was connected to a social worker who enrolled him in his state insurance plan. The insurance plan covers dialysis treatment. Mr. Jones is delighted and begins his treatment at a dialysis facility two blocks from his home and one mile from his place of employment. Mr. Jones has the perfect schedule that would allow him to make it to his dialysis appointments and not interfere with his work schedule. Mr. Jones has not missed any of his dialysis appointments. After 6 months, Mr. Jones learns that he will have to be transferred to another facility located fifteen miles from his home and work. He is not sure why he has to move and asks to speak to the facility manager to explain his situation and request that he remain at the facility. When he meets with the manager, he is asked who his insurance carrier is and immediately informed that there is limited space at the facility and new cases are being admitted daily. Mr. Jones' request is denied. He leaves the facility believing that his request was denied because of the type of insurance he had but had no proof. Since transferring to the new facility, Mr. Jones has regularly missed appointments. He has also received a written reprimand at work for absence/tardiness.

Glossary of Terms and Concepts

Counter narrative: Used to expose, analyze, and challenge deeply entrenched narratives and characterizations of racial privilege.

Dominant narrative: Used to describe the lens in which history is told from the perspective of the dominant culture.

Informed consent: Permission granted in the knowledge of the possible consequences, typically that which is given by a patient to a doctor for treatment with full knowledge of the possible risks and benefits.

Intersectionality: The interconnected nature of social categorizations such as race, class, and gender as they apply to a given individual or group, regarded as creating overlapping and interdependent systems of discrimination or disadvantage.

Social construct: It is something that exists not in objective reality, but because of human interaction. It exists because humans agree that it exists.

Jim Crow laws: Laws created by White southerners to enforce racial segregation across the South from the 1870s through the 1960s.

de facto segregation: Racial, ethnic, or other segregation resulting from societal differences between groups, as socioeconomic or political disparity, without institutionalized legislation intended to segregate.

Prison industrial complex: A term we use to describe the overlapping interests of government and industry that use surveillance, policing, and imprisonment as solutions to economic, social, and political problems.

References

Abelson, J. S., Symer, M. M., Yeo, H. L., Butler, P. D., Dolan, P. T., Moo, T. A., & Watkins, A. C. (2018). Surgical time out: our counts are still short on racial diversity in academic surgery. *The American Journal of Surgery, 215*(4), 542–548.

Ackerman-Barger, K., Boatright, D., Gonzalez-Colaso, R., Orozco, R., & Latimore, D. (2020). Seeking inclusion excellence: Understanding racial microaggressions as experienced by underrepresented medical and nursing students. *Academic Medicine, 95*(5), 758.

Allen, A., Davey, M., & Davey, A. (2010). Being examples to the Flock: The role of church leaders and African American families seeking mental health care services. *Contemporary Family Therapy: An International Journal, 32*(2), 117–134.

Almond, A. L. (2019). Measuring racial microaggression in medical practice. *Ethnicity & Health, 24*(6), 589–606.

Alsan, M., Garrick, O., & Graziani, G. (2019). Does diversity matter for health? Experimental evidence from Oakland. *American Economic Review, 109*(12), 4071–4111.

American Cancer Society. (2019). *Cancer facts and figures for African American 2019–2021* (p. 2019). American Cancer Society.

Arias, E., Escobedo, L. A., Kennedy, J., Fu, C., & Cisewski, J. (2018). U.S. small-area life expectancy estimates project: Methodology and results summary. National Center for Health Statistics. *Vital Health Stat 2*(181).

Armstrong, K., Ravenell, K. L., McMurphy, S., & Putt, M. (2007). Racial/ethnic differences in physician distrust in the United States. *American Journal of Public Health, 97*(7), 1283–1289. https://doi.org/10.2105/AJPH.2005.080762Objectives. Accessed 4 Mar 2021.

Association of American Medical Colleges. (2015). *Altering the course: Black males in medicine*. Association of American Medical Colleges.

Association of American Medical Colleges. (2017). U.S. Medical School Faculty. Available at https://www.aamc.org/data/facultyroster/reports/486050/usmsf17.html. Accessed 31 Dec 2018.

Bhatnagar, V., Diaz, S., & Bucur, P. A. (2020). The need for more mentorship in medical school. *Cureus, 12*(5).

Blocker, D. E., Romocki, L. S., Thomas, K. B., Jones, B. L., Jackson, E. J., Reid, L., & Campbell, M. K. (2006). Knowledge, beliefs and barriers associated with prostate cancer prevention and screening behaviors among African-American men. *Journal of the National Medical Association, 98*(8), 1286–1295.

Boulware, L. E., Cooper, L. A., Ratner, L. E., LaVeist, T. A., & Powe, N. R. (2003). Race and trust in the health care system. *Public Health Reports, 118*(4), 358–365.

Brandt, A. (1978). Racism and research: The case of the Tuskegee Syphilis study. *The Hastings Center Report, 8*(6), 21–29. https://doi.org/10.2307/3561468

Centers for Disease Control and Prevention. (2019). National Center for Injury Prevention and Control. Retrieved from https://www.cdc.gov/violenceprevention

Centers for Disease Control and Prevention. (2021). Summary health statistics: National health interview survey. Retrieved From: https://minorityhealth.hhs.gov/omh/browse.aspx?lvl=4&lvlid=28#:~:text=African%20Americans%20are%2050%20percent,compared%20to%20non%2DHispanic%20whites

Chatters, L. M., Taylor, R. J., Lincoln, K. D., Nguyen, A., & Joe, S. (2011). Church-based social support and suicidality among African Americans and Black Caribbeans. *Archives of Suicide Research, 15*(4), 337–353.

Chisholm, L. P., Jackson, K. R., Davidson, H. A., Churchwell, A. L., Fleming, A. E., & Drolet, B. C. (2020). Evaluation of racial microaggressions experienced during medical school training and the effect on medical student education and burnout: A validation study. *Journal of the National Medical Association, 113*, 310–314.

Cohen, C. J. (1999). *The boundaries of blackness: AIDS and the breakdown of Black politics*. University of Chicago Press.

Collins, W. L., & Perry, A. R. (2015). Black men's perspectives on the role of the Black Church in healthy relationship promotion and family stability. *Social Work and Christianity, 42*(4).

Craigie, T., Ames, G., & Kimble, C. (2020). *Conviction, imprisonment, and lost earnings: How involvement with the criminal justice system deepens inequality*. Available at https://www.brennancenter.org/sites/default/files/2020-09/EconomicImpactReport_pdf.pdf

Delgado, R., Stefancic, J., & Harris, A. (2017). *Critical race theory: An introduction* (3rd ed.). New York University Press.

Forrester-Anderson, I. T. (2005). Prostate cancer screening perceptions, knowledge and behaviors among African American men: Focus group findings. *Journal of Health Care for the Poor and Underserved, 16*(4), 22–30.

Fowler-Brown, A., Ashkin, E., Corbie-Smith, G., Thaker, S., & Pathman, D. E. (2006). Perception of racial barriers to health care in the rural South. *Journal of Health Care for the Poor and Underserved, 17*(1), 86–100.

Frakt, A. (2020). Bad medicine: The harm that comes from racism. The upshot: The new health care. *New York Times*, 1/13. https://www.nytimes.com/2020/01/13/upshot/bad-medicine-the-harm-that-comes-from-racism.html. Accessed 11 Apr 2021.

Gadson, S. (2006). The third world health status of Black American males. *Journal of the National Medical Association, 98*, 488–491.

Gilbert, K. L., Ray, R., Siddiqi, A., Shetty, S., Baker, E. A., Elder, K., & Griffith, D. M. (2016). Visible and invisible trends in Black men's health: Pitfalls and promises for addressing racial, ethnic, and gender inequities in health. *Annual Review of Public Health, 37*, 295–311. https://doi.org/10.1146/annurev-publhealth-032315-021556

Gillborn, D. (2006). Rethinking White supremacy: Who counts in 'WhiteWorld'. *Ethnicities, 6*(3), 318–340.

Gillborn, D., & Ladson-Billings, G. (2010). Critical race theory. *International Encyclopedia of Education, 6*, 341–347.

Griffith, D. M., Ellis, K. R., & Allen, J. O. (2013). An intersectional approach to social determinants of stress for African American men: Men's and Women's perspectives. *American Journal of Men's Health, 7*(4 Suppl), 19S–30S. https://doi.org/10.1177/1557988313480227

Hadinger, M. A. (2017). Underrepresented minorities in medical school admissions: A qualitative study. *Teaching and Learning in Medicine, 29*(1), 31–41.

Harris, C. I. (1993). Whiteness as property. *Harvard law review*, 1707–1791. https://doi.org/10.2307/1341787.

Holzer, H. (2021, March 1). *Why are employment rates so low among Black men?* Brookings Institution. Available at https://www.brookings.edu/research/why-are-employment-rates-so-low-among-black-men/

Jackson, J. S., & Knight, K. M. (2006). Race and self-regulatory health behaviors: The role of the stress response and the HPA axis. In K. W. Schaie & L. L. Carstensten (Eds.), *Social structure, aging and self-regulation in the elderly* (pp. 189–240). Springer.

Jindal, T., Kachroo, N., Sammon, J., Dalela, D., Sood, A., Vetterlein, M. W., … & Abdollah, F. (2017, July). Racial differences in prostate-specific antigen–based prostate cancer screening: state-by-state and region-by-region analyses. In *Urologic oncology: Seminars and original investigations* (Vol. 35, No. 7, pp. 460-e9). Elsevier.

Ladson-Billings, G. (1998). Just what is critical race theory and what's it doing in a nice field like education? *International Journal of Qualitative Studies in Education, 11*, 7–24.

Laurencin, C. T., & Murray, M. (2017). An American crisis: The lack of black men in medicine. *Journal of Racial and Ethnic Health Disparities, 4*(3), 317–321.

Lincoln, K. D., Taylor, R. J., Watkins, D. C., & Chatters, L. M. (2011). Correlates of Psychological Distress and Major Depressive DisorderAmong African American Men. *Research on Social Work Practice, 21*(3), 278–288. https://doi.org/10.1177/1049731510386122

Mahal, B. A., Chen, Y. W., Muralidhar, V., Mahal, A. R., Choueiri, T. K., Hoffman, K. E., … Nguyen, P. L. (2017). Racial disparities in prostate cancer outcome among prostate-specific antigen screening eligible populations in the United States. *Annals of Oncology, 28*(5), 1098–1104.

National Center for Health Statistics. (2019). *Health, United States, 2019*. https://doi.org/10.15620/cdc:100685.externalicon

National Urban League. (2007). *The state of Black America 2007: Portrait of the Black male.* New York: Beckham Publications Group, Inc.

Pharr, J. R., Moonie, S., & Bungum, T.J. (2012). The impact of unemployment on mental and physical health, access to health care and health risk behaviors. *International Scholarly Research Notices Public Health*, 1–7. Available at https://www.hindawi.com/archive/2012/483432/

Plowden, K., & Young, A. (2003). Sociostructural factors influencing health behaviors of urban African American men. *Journal of National Black Nurses Association, 14*, 45–50.

Powell, W., Adams, L. B., Cole-Lewis, Y., Agyemang, A., & Upton, R. D. (2016). Masculinity and race-related factors as barriers to health help-seeking among African American men. *Behavioral Medicine (Washington, D.C.), 42*(3), 150–163. https://doi.org/10.1080/08964289.2016.1165174. Accessed 26 Mar 2021

Powell, W., Richmond, J., Mohottige, D., Yen, I., Joslyn, A., & Corbie-Smith, G. (2019). Medical mistrust, racism, and delays in preventive health screening among African-American men.

Behavioral medicine (Washington, D.C.), 45(2), 102–117. https://doi.org/10.1080/0896428 9.2019.1585327

Pullano, M. (2021). Prisoners face severe Covid risks without federal vaccine priority, *Courtroom News*. Available at https://www.courthousenews.com/ prisoners-face-severe-covid-risks-without-federal-vaccine-priority/

Rao, V., & Flores, G. (2007). Why aren't there more African-American physicians? A qualitative study and exploratory inquiry of African-American students' perspectives on careers in medicine. *Journal of the National Medical Association, 99*(9), 986–993.

Ravenell, J. E., Whitaker, E. E., & Johnson, W. E., Jr. (2008). According to him: Barriers to healthcare among African-American men. *Journal of the National Medical Association, 100*(10), 1153–1160. https://doi.org/10.1016/s0027-9684(15)31479-6

Roberts, S. E., Shea, J. A., Sellers, M., Butler, P. D., & Kelz, R. R. (2020). Pursuing a career in academic surgery among African American medical students. *The American Journal of Surgery, 219*(4), 598–603.

Robinson, M. A., Jones-Eversley, S., Moore, S. E., Ravenell, J., & Adedoyin, A. C. (2018). Black Male Mental Health and the Black Church: Advancing a Collaborative Partnership and Research Agenda. *Journal of religion and health, 57*(3), 1095–1107. https://doi.org/10.1007/ s10943-018-0570-x

Rose, L., Kim, M., Dennison, C., & Hill, M. (2000). The context of adherence for African Americans with high blood pressure. *Journal of Advanced Nursing, 32*, 587–594.

Rotenstein, L. S., Reede, J. Y., & Jena, A. B. (2021). Addressing workforce diversity—A quality-improvement framework. *New England Journal of Medicine, 384*(12), 1083–1086.

Rowland, M., & Isaac-Savage, E. (2014). As I see it: A study of African American Pastors' views on health and health education in the Black Church. *Journal of Religion and Health, 53*(4), 1091–1101.

Royster, M. O., Richmond, A., Eng, E., & Margolis, L. (2006). Hey brother, how's your health? A focus group analysis of the health and health-related concerns of African American Men in a southern city in the United States. *Men and Masculinities, 8*(4), 389–404.

Sellers, S. L., Bonham, V., Neighbors, H. W., & Amell, J. W. (2009). Effects of racial discrimination and health behaviors on mental and physical health of middle-class AfricanAmerican men. *Health education & behavior: the official publication of the Society for Public Health Education, 36*(1), 31–44. https://doi.org/10.1177/1090198106293526

Serota, D. P., Rosenberg, E. S., Thorne, A. L., Sullivan, P. S., & Kelley, C. F. (2019). Lack of health insurance is associated with delays in PrEP initiation among young black men who have sex with men in Atlanta, US: A longitudinal cohort study. *Journal of the International AIDS Society, 22*(10).

Smith, T. B., & Silva, L. (2011). Ethnic identity and personal well-being of people of color: a meta-analysis. *Journal of counseling psychology, 58*(1), 42.

Stuart, A. (2019). *Prostate cancer in African American men.* https://www.webmd.com/ prostate-cancer/features/prostate-cancer-african-american-men

Taylor, E., Gillborn, D., & Ladson-Billings, G. (Eds.). (2009). *Foundations of critical race theory in education.* Routledge.

Thomas, L. A., Balon, R., Beresin, E. V., Coverdale, J., Brenner, A. M., Louie, A. K. & Roberts, L. W. (2019). *Recruitment of Black men and women into academic psychiatry.*

Thurmond, V. B., & Cregler, L. L. (1999). Why students drop out of the pipeline to health professions careers: A follow-up of gifted minority high school students. *Academic Medicine: Journal of the Association of American Medical Colleges, 74*(4), 448–451.

Vince, R. A., Scarpato, K. R., & Klausner, A. P. (2020). Fighting the 'other pandemic'—Systemic racism in urology. *Nature Reviews Urology*, 1–2.

Walker, K. O., Moreno, G., & Grumbach, K. (2012). The association among specialty, race, ethnicity, and practice location among California physicians in diverse specialties. *Journal of the National Medical Association, 104*(1–2), 46–52.

Walker, N., Bryce J., & Black, R.E. (2007). "Interpreting Health Statistics for Policymaking: The Story Behind The Headlines." *The Lancet, 369*(9565), 956–963.

Warner, D. F., & Hayward, M. D. (2006). Early-life origins of the race gap in men's mortality. *Journal of Health and Social Behavior, 47*(3), 209–226. https://doi.org/10.1177/002214650604700302

Watkins, D. C., Allen, J. O., Goodwill, J. R., & Noel, B. (2017). Strengths and weaknesses of the Young Black Men, Masculinities, and Mental Health (YBMen) Facebook project. *American Journal of Orthopsychiatry, 87*(4), 392.

Watson, J. (2014). Young African American males: Barriers to access to health care. *Journal of Human Behavior in the Social Environment, 24*(8), 1004–1009.

Whitaker, K. M., Jacobs, D. R., Kershaw, K.N., Demmer, R.T., Booth, J.N., Carson, A.P., Lewis, C.E., Goff, D.C., Lloyd-Jones, D.M., Gordon-Larsen, P., & Kiefe, C.I. (2018). Racial Disparities in Cardiovascular Health Behaviors: The Coronary Artery Risk Development in Young Adults Study. *American Journal of Preventive Medicine, 55*(1), 63–71. https://doi.org/10.1016/j.amepre.2018.03.017

Whetten, K., Leserman, J., Whetten, R., Ostermann, J., Thielman, N., Swartz, M., & Stangl, D. (2006). Exploring lack of trust in care providers and the government as a barrier to health service use. *American Journal of Public Health, 96*(4), 716–721.

Williams, D. R. (2003). The health of men: Structured inequalities and opportunities. *American Journal of Public Health, 93*(5), 724–731. https://doi.org/10.2105/ajph.93.5.724

Shonda K. Lawrence, PhD, LMSW, MS, is Associate Professor of Social Work and currently serves as Director of the PhD Program and Center for Children and Families at Clark Atlanta University in Atlanta, Georgia. Her research interests include child welfare, the impact of parental incarceration on children and families, African American fatherhood, and data science. She teaches courses in research, data science, social welfare policy, and cultural diversity. Dr. Lawrence has also received foundation, state, and federal funding to conduct research. She has several peer-reviewed journal articles, book chapters, and has presented at numerous juried conferences.

Jerry Watson, PhD, LCSW, MBA, is an assistant professor and coordinator of the Bachelor of Social Work program at the University of Memphis in Tennessee. Jerry taught sociology and psychology at DePaul University, group work at Aurora University in Chicago, and a variety of social work courses at the bachelor's, master's, and doctoral levels at Jackson State University, Mississippi Valley State University, the University of Mississippi, and Rust College. Jerry currently teaches and is the faculty lead at the University of Memphis for Social Work Practice in Community and Organizations. Dr. Watson is a scholar-activist and generalist practitioner. Jerry has over 50 years of combined experience in teaching, working in a variety of community clinical positions, and leading health and wellness programs and initiatives targeting African American men and boys. Dr. Watson's community experience and scholarship spans broadly across community topics including the following domains with a social justice lens: offender re-entry support, affordable housing, community organizing, business development, asset-based community development, cultural activism, youth and family wellness, crime and safety, community violence intervention and prevention, trauma-informed care, the "digital divide," race, culture, and poverty.

Kristie Lipford, PhD, is a medical sociologist specializing in health disparities and clinical research. Currently, she is an assistant professor in the Health Equity and Urban Studies programs at Rhodes College in Memphis, Tennessee. Her research broadly examines health behaviors, urban health services, and the socio-cultural determinants of health. Dr. Lipford's past studies have highlighted the role of psychosocial factors and medical mistrust on African American health behaviors. Her most recent work focuses on women's health and the integration of birth doulas in hospital-based maternity care. At Rhodes, she teaches Research Methods in Health Disparities, Social Statistics, and Medical Sociology.

Nathaniel Currie, DSW, MSW, LCSW, is an assistant professor at Clark Atlanta University, School of Social Work, in Atlanta, Georgia, and adjunct professor in Simmons University, Doctor of Social Work program, in Boston, Massachusetts. He has extensive post-master's practice experience in behavioral health, HIV, LGBTQ issues, men's issues, and community empowerment. He received his DSW from the University of Pennsylvania. He conducts research on trauma, health issues, resiliency, and healing in men. Dr. Currie regularly writes, presents, consults on curriculum, and speaks nationally on the application of Critical Race lens and DEIPAR (diversity, equity, inclusion, intersectionality, power analysis, anti-racist) in social work and other helping professions.

Malik Cooper, LSW, is the Director of the Counseling and Social Work Department at KIPP Atlanta Collegiate High School in Georgia. He is also a fourth-year, full-time PhD student and teaching assistant at Whitney M. Young Jr. School of Social Work at Clark Atlanta University in Georgia. Mr. Cooper received his Master of Social Work degree from the University of Pennsylvania. He is an experienced professional in Clinical Counseling and Social Work administration with a demonstrated history of working in the social services and mental healthcare industry. His research interests focus on best practices for African American youth using a trauma-informed care approach.

Chapter 12
Advocacy, Politics, and the Sporting World's Responses to Racial Unrest

Dewey M. Clayton ⓘ, **Sharon D. Jones-Eversley** ⓘ, **and Sharon E. Moore** ⓘ

Background to Black Social Movements in America

The need for racial equity in America is not a new phenomenon. Nor are Black activism and Black social movements. In this chapter, Black social movements are defined as mobilized abolitionist groups of any size engaged in various forms of Black emancipation activism (Harbour, 2020). The Black emancipation activism efforts advance the humanization, health, wellness, prosperity, and justice for persons of African descent (Grills et al., 2016; Guinier & Torres, 2014). From the African slave John Bunch's 1639 failed runaway attempt, Gabriel Prosser's rebellion attempt in 1800, or Nat Turner's 1831 revolt, Black emancipation activists have influenced, strategized, mobilized, or revolted in protest of Black inequality, oppression, and racial injustice impacting persons of African descent (Degler, 1959; Greenberg, 2003; Sidbury & James, 1997). For over 402 years, Black social movements actualized through Black emancipation activism have existed in America.

D. M. Clayton (✉)
Department of Political Science, University of Louisville, Louisville, KY, USA
e-mail: d.clayton@louisville.edu

S. D. Jones-Eversley
Department of Family Studies & Community Development, Towson University, Towson, MD, USA
e-mail: sjoneseversley@towson.edu

S. E. Moore
Raymond A. Kent School of Social Work and Family Science, University of Louisville, Louisville, KY, USA
e-mail: sharon.moore2@louisville.edu

© The Author(s), under exclusive license to Springer Nature
Switzerland AG 2022
Y. D. Dyson et al. (eds.), *Black Men's Health*,
https://doi.org/10.1007/978-3-031-04994-1_12

Critical Race Theory

In this chapter, the authors will use critical race theory (CRT) to: (1) explore the aspects of the Black social movement during the slavery-antebellum eras led by Black slave-athletes turned activists Isaac Murphy and Tom Molineaux, (2) examine the social and political transformations of the Black social movement to the twentieth-century Civil Rights Movement, and (3) reflect upon the state of race relations in America during the twenty-first century and the era of Black Lives Matter.

Viewed as an academic or intellectual social movement, critical race theory (CRT) was developed by Derrick Bell, a civil rights attorney and legal scholar (Bell, 1995). CRT operationalizes race, ethnicity, and racism as socially constructed hierarchies. It provides a social-scientific approach to explaining the cultural oppressiveness of inequality, privilege, power, and dominance in a xenophobic society (Delgado & Stefancic, 2005; Gilmore, 1995).

Critical race theorist Cheryl Harris adds a theoretical approach to "whiteness" as property – the ultimate property that white people alone can possess. She draws an analogy to the white skin color some Americans can possess as being akin to owning a piece of property. It gives privilege to the owner that a renter (or a person of color) would not be afforded (Harris, 1995). Therefore, CRT is an ideal lens to examine Black emancipation activism, the Civil Rights Movement in the twentieth century, and the status of race relations in America at the dawn of the twenty-first century. CRT allows us to understand the continuation of the Black liberation movement in America in the era of the Black Lives Matter Movement and the response to the racial violence in America, and renewed activism on the part of Black athletes.

Blacks and Sports Before the Twentieth Century

Since 1619, when American colonialists at Old Point Comfort in Jamestown, Virginia, stole African slaves from a Portuguese ship, African slaves and their children were legally viewed as the property of their slave owners (Thornton, 1998). Black slavery in America was a legalized chattel system. This system dehumanized, traumatized, and monetarized Black bodies through physical, sexual, and psychological abuses (Foster, 2011; Johnson, 2018).

Just as there were well-known Black abolitionists for racial justice, such as Harriet Tubman, Frederick Douglass, Henry Box Brown, etc., there were also Black slave-athlete activists. In the sporting world, the Black slave-athletes Isaac Murphy and Tom Molineaux protested the racialized oppression against Black slaves. Their emancipation activism led to contractual maneuvering that resulted in Tom Molineaux purchasing his freedom from slavery (Furer, 1994). Like Molineaux, Isaac Murphy was also born into slavery. Murphy was a well-paid jockey and a three-time Kentucky Derby winner (Mooney, 2017).

Particularly for enslaved Black men, enslavers, mostly White, monetized Black male bodies in betting sports-related competitions like boxing, wrestling, and horseracing (Rhoden, 2006; Gilmore, 1995; Zallen, 2015). In boxing and wrestling, these so-called *bare-knuckled fights* usually ended in the enslaved Black person seriously injuring or killing his enslaved Black opponent (Dokosi, 2019). And in horse racing, the enslaved Black jockeys were dehumanized and viewed as property and whipped, like the horses they rode (Campbell, 2015). Although some research justifies the sport pawning of Black male slaves as recreational outlets to ease the brutality of slave life, living a shackled and chattel existence is far from easing the cruel and inhumane nature of slavery (Griffith, 2010; Miller et al., 2018).

Before notable social justice activists in sports in the twentieth century, like Jack Johnson, Muhammad Ali, Tommie Smith, John Carlos, and Colin Kaepernick, began speaking out against racial injustice, Black slave-athletes turned activists jockey Isaac Murphy and boxer Tom Molineaux predated them all. (Coombs et al., 2020; McCaffrey, 2020; Teresa, 2015).

After the Civil War ended, America went through the period known as Reconstruction in the South. It was an attempt by the national government to bestow the full rights of citizenship on the newly freed enslaved Americans. In 1865, Congress abolished slavery with passage of the thirteenth Amendment, followed three years later by the fourteenth Amendment, which granted automatic citizenship to anyone born in America and bestowed on them the "equal protection of the laws." Finally, in 1870, Congress passed the fifteenth Amendment, which prohibited states from denying anyone the right to vote based on race, color, or "previous condition of servitude." When federal troops were withdrawn from the South after the Hayes-Tilden Comprise of 1876, Reconstruction ended, and the South reverted to its antebellum ways, denying Blacks their newly gained rights. Blacks were reduced to a state of peonage in the South. In *Plessy v. Ferguson* (1896), the US Supreme Court handed down the doctrine of "separate but equal," which said the state could require separation of the races if it provided Blacks with equal accommodations to those given to whites (Sitkoff, 2008). However, during the late nineteenth and early twentieth centuries, Black and White athletes competed against one another in football, basketball, horse racing, and other sports. But as Black athletes began to dominate these sports, interracial competition was prohibited. Black athletes would be banned from all professional sports in America until the 1940s (Walter, 1996). Whites justified their fear of losing to Black athletes by fabricating stories that Blacks were inferior athletes both mentally and physically (Walter, 1996).

The Civil Rights Movement

In the years preceding World War II, Black athletes in America were not allowed to breach the color line and were restricted from competition in professional sports. Only in the Olympics, because of its international nature, were Blacks allowed to compete (Walter, 1996). After Black heavyweight boxing champion, Jack Johnson was defeated in 1915, white boxers refused to fight a Black boxer until Joe Louis fought Jimmy Braddock in 1936 to become the heavyweight champion of the world. Black track and field star Jesse Owens, who in the 1936 Olympics in Berlin, Germany, won four gold medals and shattered Hitler's myth of Aryan superiority. Nonetheless, he was not invited to the White House to shake hands with President Roosevelt or sent a congratulatory telegram (Zirin, 2008).

By the mid-1930s, civil rights had become a major national concern in the Black community. Civil rights organizations such as the National Association for the Advancement of Colored People (NAACP), founded in 1909, had begun pursuing legal challenges to end discrimination in voting rights, housing, and school segregation. The Congress of Racial Equality (CORE), founded in 1942, began experimenting with nonviolent direct action to protest Jim Crow segregation in interstate travel. Additionally, Blacks had gained entrance into the American Federation of Labor, and other labor unions, and these organizations began exerting additional pressure on public institutions to treat Blacks as equal citizens (Walter, 1996). Blacks, plagued by powerlessness, were unable to attack segregation and fight for equal opportunity. World War II put a stop to Black protests – the nation demanded unity and winning the war at all costs (Sitkoff, 2008).

However, with the advent of World War II, the attitude of Blacks in America began to change. Black GIs fought abroad to make the world safe for democracy and returned home to a segregated America determined to fight racism and demand a better deal (Williams, 1988). By the mid-1940s, Blacks began to integrate professional football (Kenny Washington and Woody Strode) and professional baseball (Jackie Robinson), and college athletics by the beginning of the 1950s. Journalist Howard Bryant noted in his book *The Heritage*, that of all the African American employees in America's history, it is the Black athletes who have been the most influential and most important. He stated the African American intellectuals: the thinkers – the doctors, the lawyers, and the scientists were roadblocked by segregation. It was the Black athlete who was first allowed into mainstream America – the first to gain entrance into White universities and to join the White professional sports leagues (Bryant, 2018).

In 1954, the struggle for Black equality gained fresh momentum in the *Brown v. Board of Education* Supreme Court ruling mandating public school desegregation. The *Brown* decision gave renewed confidence to Blacks in pursuit of their constitutional rights to full citizenship and furthered their desire to participate in interracial sporting events (Walter, 1996). In 1955, the Civil Rights Movement began in Montgomery, Alabama, with the bus boycott led by Dr. Martin Luther King. Their weapon of protest was nonviolent civil disobedience. In 1960, the Student Nonviolent Coordinating Committee (SNCC) formed, and college students (both Black and white) began sit-ins at Whites-only lunch counters across America (Williams, 1988). Jackie Robinson went on a speaking tour to raise money for SNCC, and he and other Black athletes began encouraging Blacks to register to vote (Zirin, 2008). In 1963, Dr. Martin Luther King delivered his famous "I have a dream" speech on the steps of the Lincoln Memorial in Washington, D.C., to a multi-racial crowd of over 250,000 Americans. In 1964, Congress passed the Civil Rights Act into law, banning segregation in all public facilities and prohibiting discrimination in employment. In 1965, Johnson would sign the Voting Rights Act into law, mandating that no Americans could be denied access to the ballot box. However, many Black athletes were not speaking out against racial injustices at that time. As trailblazers, Black athletes were aware of the racial indignities of segregation in America (especially in the South) from not being able to stay in the same hotels as their White teammates, or dine at the same restaurants, to being subjected to racial epithets by white fans. However, much of their protest was met then, as today, with the reply, "Shut up and play ball."

Things would soon begin to change. By 1967, Muhammad Ali, the heavyweight boxing champion of the world, had been stripped of his heavyweight title for refusing to be inducted into the Vietnam War as a "conscientious objector." His application was rejected, and he was facing charges of draft-dodging. Jim Brown, a Cleveland Browns running back, who recently retired as the all-time leading rusher in the National Football League, invited Ali and a group of the most talented Black athletes in the country to a meeting in Cleveland, now known as the "Cleveland Summit."

They were called to decide whether to support Ali and discuss what impact Ali's decision would have on other Black athletes and on Black America. Those in attendance that day included Washington Redskins running back Bobby Mitchell, Boston Celtics center Bill Russell, UCLA center Lewis Alcindor, and Cleveland attorney Carl Stokes. Later that year, Stokes would become the first African American mayor of a major city in the United States (Eig, 2017).

In 1968, Harry Edwards, a Black sociology graduate student and former track athlete at San Diego State University, organized the Olympic Project for Human Rights (OPHR), calling for a boycott by African Americans of the 1968 Summer Olympics in Mexico City. The main goal was to expose how the United States used African American athletes to portray a false image of race relations at home and abroad (Zirin, 2012, p. 2). They had four central demands, most notably to restore Muhammad Ali's boxing title. The OPHR's emancipation activism and boycott led to the iconic, Black-gloved Black Power salute on the second day of the Olympics by two of the top three finishers in the 200-meter race: gold medalist Tommie Smith and bronze medalist John Carlos. The silver medalist Australian Peter Norman wore an OPHR patch on his chest to show solidarity with the others. It was a defining moment in the history of sports and protest. Smith and Carlos wore no shoes to protest Black poverty in America and beads and scarves to protest the lynching of African Americans in the United States. Both were suspended from the summer games, and all three sprinters' Olympic careers were effectively over (Zirin, 2012, p. 3).

In an interview given to *People* magazine in 2014, President Obama praised basketball star LeBron James and other athletes who were protesting the killing of unarmed African Americans by police officers. Obama noted, James and others were following a rich tradition of athletes speaking out, especially during the volatile 1960s. He said, "We forget the role that Muhammad Ali, Arthur Ashe and Bill Russell played in raising consciousness" (Jackson, 2014, p. 1). Muhammad Ali and

Arthur Ashe could not have been more opposite in personalities (one brash, the other soft-spoken), but both were transformative sports figures whose impact off the court and ring rivaled their athletic prowess.

Ashe grew up in segregated Richmond, Virginia, where Jim Crow laws of the day would not allow him to play against white opponents in the state. He would go on to win both the US Amateur Open and the US Open (one of the four major Grand Slam events in tennis) in 1968. Ashe would protest racism both at home and abroad. He was a Pan-Africanist and took an active role in the anti-apartheid protest against the racist practices of South Africa. Some questioned his authenticity. Bryant said that Harry Edwards felt Ashe was an "Uncle Tom" because he did not participate in the civil rights protests in the 1960s. Ashe, however, was no Uncle Tom. He demanded self-industriousness and American acknowledgment of institutional racism. Ashe remarked after winning Wimbledon in 1975, "I know what it's like to be stepped on. So, I know what it's like also to see some Black hero do well in the face of adversity" (Bryant, 2018, p. 133).

Beginning with the decade of the 1970s and for 50 years, activism on the part of Black athletes completely disappeared. Buffalo Bills star running back O.J. "The Juice" Simpson redirected African American athletes from "Black issues to green issues," and it opened a world of financial opportunities for the Black athlete. In 1975, Hertz rental car company made Simpson the first African American to lead an advertising campaign and made him the most visible Black athlete in team sports – and it made Simpson a superstar. Simpson proved that marketing opportunities were now opening for Black athletes, who had a certain appeal to Whites by being willing to cool the politics and the anger (Bryant, 2018).

As salaries and sports revenues grew in the 1980s and 1990s, Black activism remained on the sidelines. By the 1990s, due to the globalization of the National Basketball Association, Michael Jordan's brand reached millions around the world. Jordan's endorsements (everyone wants to be like Mike) would make him the first billionaire athlete of any race. In 1996, Black pro golfer Tiger Woods signed a $40 million endorsement deal with Nike at the age of 20. Civil rights activist Al Sharpton would proclaim, "In the 1980s and '90s, racial incidents flared up throughout New York City from Howard Beach, Bensonhurst, Amadou Diallo, through Albert Louima, there was no support from the athletes" (Bryant, 2018, p. 91).

Police Brutality and Mass Incarceration

The protests in the South during the Civil Rights Movement led to meaningful civil rights legislation (see previous section). Northern Blacks were aware of how southern Blacks gained major civil rights victories by using nonviolent, peaceful protest. Tired of living in squalid conditions in urban slums and ghettos of the North, they were eager for change too. As a result, they took to the streets to protest a system that did not allow them to share in the opportunities and benefits that most northern Whites enjoyed (Sitkoff, 2008). Beginning in the mid-1960s, urban rioting erupted in Los Angeles, Newark, Detroit, and in more than 160 other cities in Black and poor inner-city neighborhoods across America. They were met with police brutality.

A report by the Kerner Commission appointed to investigate the causes of the civil unrest said our nation is moving toward two societies: one Black, one White – separate and unequal. After the report was issued, more rioting broke out after the assassination of Dr. Martin Luther King. Shortly thereafter, Congress passed the Fair Housing Act, outlawing discrimination in housing. Richard Nixon was elected president in 1968 on a "law and order" platform, which included running television ads calling on voters to reject the lawlessness of civil rights activists and embrace order in the United States (Alexander, 2010; Katel, 2018).

Beginning in the 1970s, the country underwent a major structural shift in the US economy. Labor-intensive manufacturing plants, including textile mills in the South, began moving to Mexico and overseas to Asia. The impact of globalization and deindustrialization had a devastating effect on Black inner-city neighborhoods. Additionally, many good-paying blue-collar jobs left the central cities across America and migrated to the White suburbs (Katel, 2018). Many Blacks were trapped in ghettos, isolated and jobless. Legal scholar Michelle Alexander would note, "the decline in legitimate employment opportunities among inner city residents increased incentives to sell drugs – most notably crack cocaine" (Alexander, 2010, p. 50).

During the 1980s, urban crime exploded due to crack cocaine. In 1992, rioting broke out for five days after the acquittal of three police officers – stoked by years of racial and economic inequality – charged with assault and the use of excessive force in a videotaped beating of Rodney King, an African American, after a high-speed chase through Los Angeles County. In 1994, Congress responded to the increased urban crime by passing the largest anti-crime bill in history, requiring life imprisonment without parole after three violent or drug-trafficking convictions and allotting $10 billion for prisons. States followed with similar measures. As a result, the prison population across America due to homicide deaths and drug-trafficking offenses soared. By 2000, 10% of all Black males aged 25–29 years were incarcerated (Katel, 2018). Michelle Alexander has referred to racial profiling and the targeting of drug enforcement in African American communities as "the new Jim Crow" (Alexander, 2010). In the two decades since, the issues of police misconduct, racial bias, and the mass incarceration of Black males have grabbed the national spotlight.

State Violence Against Black Bodies and the Rise of Black Lives Matter

Trauma is an ever-present reality in the lived experiences of Black Americans. By definition, trauma is "an exposure to an extraordinary experience that presents a physical or psychological threat to oneself or others and generates a reaction of helplessness and fear" (Levenson, 2017, p. 105). For more than 400 years, Black people in the U.S. have suffered needless and profound pain as a result of white-racist supremacy, the ensuing systematic oppression and inequalities, and the resultant anti-Black sentiment that so pervasively affects them in every area of their lives. The legacy of the horrific mistreatment they endured during the era of U.S. slavery, as discussed earlier, rarely acknowledged by White America, is compounded by police shootings of unarmed Black men and women. Since 2015, roughly 5000 Black people have been shot and killed by an on-duty police officer *(The Washington Post*, 2020). Although Black people make up 13% of the U.S. population, they are killed by police twice as often as White Americans. Since the U.S. slave era, there have been countless police killings of unarmed Black people, such as Jonny Gammage, Tanisha N. Anderson, Walter Lamar Scott, Freddie Gray, Antwon Rose, Sandra Bland, and Terence Crutcher. In 2020, George Floyd was killed by a White police officer who kept his knee on Mr. Floyd's neck for at least 9 min and 29 s while Mr. Floyd gasped for air and cried out over 20 times that he could not breathe. Shortly thereafter, he became unconscious and later died (Associated Press, 2021).

There have been scores of police killings of unarmed Black people before and after Mr. Floyd's death. However, the horrific nature in which he died, which was video recorded by bystanders, precluded the public from denying the circumstances of his death and the impact of racism on the lives of Black Americans and has subsequently caused worldwide outrage and protests. The shooting of Duante Wright by a police officer occurred after Mr. Floyd's untimely death. The white police officer claimed that she mistook her revolver for a taser (BBC News, 2021). Black Lives Matter (BLM) was at the forefront of anti-racism and political activism. As a Black emancipation activism and social justice movement, BLM was founded in 2013 in response to the murder of Trayvon Martin (Simon, 2017) and helped bring international awareness and activism against white supremacy and violence inflicted on Black communities by the state and vigilantes (Black Lives Matter, n.d.).

Whether athletes play for major or minor teams, they have fans who follow them closely through social, print, or broadcast media. Those platforms substantially impact public opinion, "When athletes publicly adopt a cause, it's hard to dismiss." Because the athletes' branding and high visibility are seen as credible, the causes they take a stance on are often embraced by the public (Jude, 2020).

Black athletes use their celebrity status and platforms to protest police shootings of unarmed Black people. Colin Kaepernick, Russell Westbrook, Lebron James, and Naomi Osaka are among the most notable. In 2016, Colin Kaepernick, quarterback for the San Francisco 49ers, refused to stand for the national anthem in protest of the police killing of Black people and the oppression of all minoritized people. Instead of standing, he knelt in opposition to all forms of inequality and repression. His protest and Black emancipation activism ignited international conversations about police brutality and white privilege. Research indicates that Black Americans widely embraced his emancipation activism. Almost 80% of Black people favored his and other players' objection to the national anthem (Towler et al., 2019). Many people believe Kaepernick's protests spotlight police violence and demand justice for Black people. However, as a direct result of his activism, he was blackballed from the National Football League (NFL) and lost his job (costing him tens of millions of dollars) and his NFL career (Murray, 2018). Los Angeles Lakers player Lebron James, arguably the greatest basketball player of all time, has used his celebrity platform to highlight his political activism on voter repression and police brutality against Black males. After the death of George Floyd, he created an organization called "More than a Vote" that works toward organizing Black voters and undoing voter suppression (Bunn, 2020). James worked in conjunction with the NAACP Legal Defense Fund to enlist 40,000 poll workers through his organization. He assisted Florida residents who had felony records unrelated to murder or sexual assault in registering to vote. He also played a critical role in ensuring that 23 out of 30 National Basketball Association (NBA) teams utilized their home arenas or practice venues as voting locations (Medina, 2020). In addition to this work, most recently, he served as executive producer for the CNN documentary Dreamland about Black Wall Street (Smith, 2020). Tennis player Naomi Osaka, the world's highest-paid female athlete, exemplifies the many forms that Black emancipation activism can take.

As a result of the death of Breonna Taylor, Naomi Osaka leveraged her Black emancipation activism by bringing awareness of police brutality – particularly police brutality that killed Black people. She wore facial masks at her tennis matches that displayed the names of unarmed Black people who had been killed by police (Tandon, 2020). After George Floyd was killed, videos by NFL players insisting on change and racial justice provoked an apology by League commissioner Roger Goodell for not taking seriously the protests by Colin Kaepernick. As a result of players' calls for the leagues to work towards the betterment of Black lives, the NFL, the NBA, and other professional leagues started integrating social justice mottos on playing fields and players' uniforms. In August of 2020, professional basketball, baseball, football, and tennis organized a mass walkout in which Osaka participated protesting yet another police shooting of a Black man, Jacob Blake, in Kenosha, Wisconsin.

The political influence of Black players within the sports industry can be considered from a Marxian perspective. In a capitalist society, such as the United States, money is the primary motivator for all socio-political activity. Under this social and economic system, the primary objective is the acquisition of wealth and the accumulation of capital (Tucker, 1978). Collectively, the US sports industry is estimated to be worth $500 billion dollars, with $250 billion of that related to professional sports. This revenue figure includes television distribution, fitness, ticketing, betting, advertising, sponsorship, and merchandising. Of the most popular U.S. sports, basketball has 6% of revenue, and football has 13% (Torrenns University, 2020). Within those sports, Black players make up 74% and 59%, respectively, and 67% of professional women basketball players are Black (Santamaria & Winkleman, 2020). A key point for consideration is that Black athletes create revenue that pays for their salaries and the salaries of the coaching staff, other administrators, and a plethora of ancillary jobs and goods and services that contribute to the economy. Hence, Black players' emancipation activism can influence public opinion, law, and policymakers and have an impact on political discourse.

Summary

In 1954, the US Supreme Court issued its decision in the landmark *Brown v. Board of Education* case, which outlawed segregation in public schools across America. It served as the catalyst for the Civil Rights Movement of the 1950s and 1960s. The Civil Rights Movement renewed efforts of Blacks in this country to end the system of racial apartheid in the American South and across the nation. Civil rights activists began an attack on Jim Crow segregation by using the weapon of nonviolent, peaceful protests in the form of bus boycotts, sit-ins at segregated lunch counters in department stores, freedom rides, and marches to register Blacks to vote. The movement needed the political mobilization of Black and white Americans committed to the cause of social justice. Within five years of the March on Washington, where Dr. Martin Luther King delivered his famous "I have a dream" speech, on the Washington Mall in 1963 to a crowd of 250,000 people, Congress passed three significant civil rights laws. This legislation outlawed discrimination in all areas of public accommodation, employment, and housing. It required states to provide equal access to the polls, giving the Justice Department prior approval over southern states with any laws prohibiting Blacks from voting.

Also, by the 1950s, professional sporting teams had begun recruiting some Blacks. In the 1960s, colleges and universities across the country followed suit, but only on a limited basis, especially in the South. Black athletes suffered the indignities of racial discrimination, and their protests were largely met with the refrain: shut up and play ball. However, that would change in 1967. That year an array of Black superstar athletes met in Cleveland, Ohio, to lend support to heavyweight boxing champion Muhammad Ali. The event, now known as the "Cleveland Summit," was called to lend support to Ali, who had recently refused induction into the armed services and the Vietnam War. The next year, at the 1968 Summer Olympics, two Black medal winners in the 200-meter race raised a black-gloved, Black Power salute at the iconic medal stand to protest race relations in America and abroad. However, for roughly the next 50 years, social activism on the part of Black athletes disappeared, especially at the professional level. For nearly a half-century, Black professional athletes were too preoccupied with the amount of money they could make in salaries and corporate endorsements – and social justice issues took a back seat.

Recent events around the country have changed that attitude, however. Starting in the decade of 2010, several high-profile police shootings of unarmed Black males spawned a new social movement: Black Lives Matter. Its tactics and leadership style differ from the Civil Rights Movement; however, it is just the next iteration by Blacks in the continuing struggle for Black Liberation in America. BLM has brought national attention to police brutality and lit a spark underneath Black athletes, both at the collegiate and professional level, who have begun speaking out against police brutality and urging fellow athletes to advocate publicly for change. None has been more outspoken than Colin Kaepernick, a San Francisco 49ers professional football player who began taking a knee during the playing of the National Anthem at the beginning of each game.

On May 25, 2020, George Floyd, a resident of Minneapolis, Minnesota, was handcuffed and forced to the ground in a prone position by a Minnesota police officer. He placed his knee on Floyd's neck for approximately nine minutes and 29 seconds, and the incident was filmed by a bystander.

It was an inflection point in protest in this country. Black athletes have continued their activism and protest beyond protesting police brutality and racial injustice in the area of voting rights. The social injustice movements that civil rights activists and Black emancipation activists-athletes sought to solve over 50 years ago have endured. Black emancipation activists-athletes are stepping up to the plate, and they are active in today's Black Lives Matter movement.

Discussion Questions

1. Why do some Americans think sports and politics should be separate entities?
2. Why did Black athletes and their social activism end for almost half a century, beginning with the 1970s?
3. When Tommie Smith and John Carlos gave their iconic black-gloved, Black Power salute at the 1968 Olympic Games, who was the third individual receiving a medal and also was involved in the protest?
4. What are the historical factors that have contributed to Black athletes' political activism?
5. Will systematic racism in American sports ever diminish? If so, what will be the contributing factors?

Exercises

1. Discuss how the emancipation activism of the Black athletes of the 1960s grew out of the Civil Rights Movement in the 1950s and 1960s.
2. Discuss how the activism of Black athletes today grew out of the Black Lives Matter movement.
3. Discuss how sports-based protests continue to remain polarizing in American society.
4. Discuss how athletic activism is closely related to and grows out of larger racial-social movements.
5. Write a two-page paper on the athlete who, in your opinion, has helped to improve the lived experience for Black people. What specific actions did that person do? What were the outcomes of the action(s)?

Glossary of Terms and Concepts

Social movements: Mobilized abolitionist groups of any size engaged in various forms of Black emancipation activism.

Emancipation activism: Mobilized freedom and liberation efforts targeted to advance the humanization, health, wellness, prosperity, and justice for persons of African descent.

Critical race theory (CRT): A social-scientific approach that explains the socially constructed hierarchies of race, ethnicity, and racism. CRT provides a lens of how race, ethnicity, and racism are structurally weaponized in a xenophobic society. Xenophobic societies culturally and systemically oppress and maintain inequality, privilege, power, and dominance over marginalized groups.

New Jim Crow: Rebirth of a caste-like system in the United States, resulting in the mass incarceration of millions of Black men.

Racism: The belief that inherited physical characteristics, such as skin color, facial features, hair texture, and the like, determine behavior patterns, personality traits, or intellectual abilities. It is operationalized by discrimination and prejudice.

Black Lives Matter: This movement was founded in 2013 in response to the murder of Trayvon Martin and helped to bring international awareness and activism against White supremacy and violence inflicted on Black communities by the state and vigilantes.

References

Alexander, M. (2010). *The new Jim Crow: Mass incarceration in the age of colorblindness.* New Press.

Associated Press. (2021). Expert: Derek Chauvin never took knee off George Floyd's neck. *Politico.* Retrieved from https://www.politico.com/news/2021/04/07/derek-chauvin-george-floyd-trial-479796

BBC. (2021). Daunte Wright shooting: Officer 'mistook gun for Taser'. *BBC News.* Retrieved from https://www.bbc.com/news/world-us-canada-56724798

Bell, D. (1995). Who's afraid of critical race theory? *University of Illinois Law Review, 4,* 893–910.

Black Lives Matter. (n.d.). Retrieved from https://blacklivesmatter.com/about/

Bryant, H. (2018). *The heritage: Black athletes, a divided America, and the politics of patriotism.* Beacon Press.

Bunn, C. (2020). How Lebron James has become a leading voice for social justice in a racially divided nation. *News.* Retrieved from https://www.nbcnews.com/news/nbcblk/how-lebron-james-has-become-leading-voice-social-justice-racially-n1231391

Campbell, J. N. (2015). Race horse men: How slavery and freedom were made at the racetrack. *The International Journal of the History of Sport, 32*(2), 387–389. https://doi.org/10.1080/09523367.2014.975431

Coombs, D. S., Lambert, C. A., Cassilo, D., & Humphries, Z. (2020). Flag on the play: Colin Kaepernick and the protest paradigm. *Howard Journal of Communications, 31*(4), 317–336. https://doi.org/10.1080/10646175.2019.1567408

Degler, C. N. (1959). Slavery and the genesis of American race prejudice. *Comparative Studies in Society and History, 2*(1), 49–66. http://www.jstor.org/stable/177546

Delgado, R., & Stefancic, J. (2005). White superiority in America: Its legal legacy, its economic costs. In *The Derrick Bell reader* (pp. 27–32). New York University Press. http://www.jstor.org/stable/j.ctt9qg47z.6

Dokosi, M. E. (2019, November 21). How enslaved Blacks beating each other to near-death was a great source of entertainment and cash for white plantation owners. *Face 2 Face Africa.* https://face2faceafrica.com/article/how-enslaved-blacks-beating-each-other-to-neardeath-was-a-great-source-of-entertainment-and-cash-for-white-plantation-owners

Eig, J. (2017, June 1). The Cleveland Summit and Muhammad Ali: The true story. *Andscape.* Retrieved from https://andscape.com/features/the-cleveland-summit-muhammad-ali/

Foster, T. (2011). The sexual abuse of Black men under American slavery. *Journal of the History of Sexuality, 20*(3), 445–464. http://www.jstor.org/stable/41305880

Furer, H. B. (1994). Tom Molineaux: America's first Black sports hero. *New England Journal of History, 51*(2), 4–13.

Gilmore, A. (1995). Black athletes in an historical context: The issue of race. *Negro History Bulletin, 58*(3/4), 7–14. http://www.jstor.org/stable/44177147

Greenberg, K. S. (Ed.). (2003). *Nat Turner: A slave rebellion in history and memory*. Oxford University Press.

Griffith, J. (2010). Sports in shackles: The athletic and recreational habits of slaves on Southern plantations. *Voces Novae, 2*(1), 59–80. https://digitalcommons.chapman.edu/vocesnovae/vol2/iss1/11

Grills, C. N., Aird, E. G., & Rowe, D. (2016). Breathe, baby, breathe: Clearing the way for the emotional emancipation of Black people. *Cultural Studies ↔ Critical Methodologies, 16*(3), 333–343. https://doi.org/10.1177/1532708616634839

Guinier, L., & Torres, G. (2014). Changing the wind: Notes toward a demosprudence of law and social movements. *The Yale Law Journal, 123*(8), 2740–2804. http://www.jstor.org/stable/43617006

Harbour, J. R. (2020). *Organizing freedom: Black emancipation activism in the Civil War Midwest*. Southern Illinois University Press.

Harris, C. (1995). Whiteness as Property. In K. Crenshaw, N. Gotanda, G. Peller, & K. Thomas (Eds.), *Critical race theory: The key writings that formed the movement*. New Press.

Jackson, D. (2014), December 19). Obama: More sports stars should speak out on issues. *USA Today*, Retrieved from https://www.usatoday.com/story/theoval/2014/12/19/obama-sports-stars-lebron-james-muhammad-ali-arthur-ashe-bill-russell/20629235/

Johnson, J. M. (2018). Markup bodies Black [Life] studies and slavery [Death] studies at the digital crossroads. *Social Text, 36*(4(137)), 57–79. https://doi.org/10.1215/01642472-7145658

Jude, A. (2020, August 27), Conversations about race and equality resonate at all levels in sports—not just the big leagues. The Seattle Times. https://www.seattletimes.com/pacific-nw-magazine/the-backstory-xxxx/

Katel, P. (2018). Racial conflict. In *Issues in race and ethnicity* (Congressional quarterly researcher) (8th ed., pp. 255–280). CQ Press.

Levenson, J. (2017). Trauma-informed social work practice. *Social Work, 62*(2), 105–113. https://doi.org/10.1093/sw/swx001

McCaffrey, R. (2020). From baseball icon to crusading columnist: How Jackie Robinson used his column in the African-American Press to continue his fight for civil rights in sports. *Journalism History, 46*(3), 185–207. https://doi.org/10.1080/00947679.2020.1757345

Medina, M. (2020). LeBron James on 'More Than a Vote': 'We just wanted to educate you, enlighten you and empower you'. *USA Today*. Retrieved from https://www.usatoday.com/story/sports/nba/lakers/2020/12/08/lebron-james-more-than-a-vote-initiative-elections/6484129002/

Miller, I. K., Steinfeldt, J. A., Richter, J. G., & McKinley, M. T. (2018). Nyane: The reemergence of Black resistant masculinity through sport. *Spectrum: A Journal on Black Men, 6*(2), 65–85. https://doi.org/10.2979/spectrum.6.2.04

Mooney, K. (2017). "I Got the Horse Right Here": New directions in horseracing scholarship. *The Register of the Kentucky Historical Society, 115*(4), 645–660. Retrieved May 21, 2021, from http://www.jstor.org/stable/44981262

Murray, C. (2018). Murray's Mailbag: How much money did Colin Kaepernick cost himself with protest? *Reno Gazette-Journal*. Retrieved from https://www.rgj.com/story/sports/college/nevada/2018/08/20/murrays-mailbag-how-much-money-did-colin-kaepernick-lose-protest/1044306002/

Rhoden, W. C. (2006). *Forty million dollar slaves*. Three Rivers Press.

Santamaria, C., & Winkleman, A. (2020). *The graphic truth: Racial diversity in US professional sports*. GZERO. Retrieved from https://www.gzeromedia.com/the-graphic-truth-racial-diversity-in-us-professional-sports

Sidbury, J., & James, S. (1997). *Ploughshares into swords: Race, rebellion, and identity in Gabriel's Virginia, 1730–1810*. Cambridge University Press.

Simon, D. (2017). *Trayvon Martin's death sparked a movement that lives on five years later*. CNN. Retrieved from https://www.cnn.com/2017/02/26/us/trayvon-martin-death-anniversary/index.html

Sitkoff, H. (2008). *The struggle for Black equality*. Farrar, Straus and Giroux.

Smith, N. (2020). *LeBron James and CNN films team up for Black Wall Street documentary*. Retrieved from https://www.forbes.com/sites/nashasmith/2020/10/26/lebron-james-and-cnn-films-team-up-for-black-wall-street-documentary/?sh=16450ca73b50

Tandon, K. (2020). Top moments of 2020: Osaka's social activism sends message at US open. *US Open*. Retrieved from https://www.tennis.com/news/articles/top-moments-of-2020-osaka-s-social-activism-sends-message-at-us-open

Teresa, C. (2015). "We Needed a Booker T. Washington… and certainly a Jack Johnson": The Black Press, Johnson, and issues of representation, 1909–1915. *American Journalism, 32*(1), 23–40. https://doi.org/10.1080/08821127.2015.999539

The Washington Post. (2020). *1000 people have been shot and killed by the police in the past year*. Retrieved from https://www.washingtonpost.com/graphics/investigations/police-shootings-database/

Thornton, J. (1998). The African experience of the "20. and Odd Negroes" arriving in Virginia in 1619. *The William and Mary Quarterly, 55*(3), 421–434. https://doi.org/10.2307/2674531

Torrenns University. (2020). *Why the sports industry is booming in 2020*. Retrieved from https://www.torrens.edu.au/blog/why-sports-industry-is-booming-in-2020-which-key-playersdriving-growth#.YK_2fvlKiUk

Towler, C., Crawford, N., & Bennett, R. (2019). Shut up and play: Black athletes, protest politics, and Black political action. *Perspectives on Politics, 18*(1), 111–127.

Tucker, R. (1978). *The Marx-Engle reader* (2nd ed.). W. W. Norton.

Walter, J. (1996). *The changing status of the Black athlete in the 20ᵗʰ Century*. Retrieved from http://www.americansc.org.uk/Online/walters.htm

Williams, J. (1988). *Eyes on the prize. New York*. Penguin Books.

Zallen, J. B. (2015). [Review of the book *Race Horse Men: How Slavery and Freedom Were Made at the Racetrack*, by Katherine C. Mooney]. *Register of the Kentucky Historical Society, 113*(4), 753–754. https://doi.org/10.1353/khs.2015.0054

Zirin, D. (2008). *A people's history of sports in the United States*. The New Press.

Zirin, D. (2012, July 25). Fists of freedom: An olympic story not taught in school. *The Nation*. Retrieved from https://www.thenation.com/article/fists-freedom-olympicstory-not-taught-school/

Dewey M. Clayton, PhD, is Professor of Political Science at the University of Louisville in Kentucky. His research interests include race, law, and politics; congressional redistricting; voting rights; and social movements (specifically the Civil Rights Movement and the Black Lives Matter Movement). He is the author of the books *African Americans and the Politics of Congressional Redistricting* (Routledge) and *The Presidential Campaign of Barack Obama* (Routledge) and numerous scholarly articles. In 2016, he was the recipient of the American Political Science Association Distinguished Teaching Award.

Sharon D. Jones-Eversley, DrPH, is a tenured associate professor and social epidemiologist at Towson University in Maryland in the Department of Family Studies and Community Development. Her interdisciplinary research expertise is in social epidemiology, family science, and community capacity-building. Her advocacy and research look to better understand intergenerational disease distribution and the continuum of disease-related morbidities that adversely affect Black families and communities. She is concerned about the disproportionate diminished health outcomes, high morbidity and mortality rates, deprivation, injustice, violence, and premature deaths impacting Black families and communities.

Sharon E. Moore, PhD, is Professor of Social Work at the Raymond A. Kent School of Social Work at the University of Louisville in Kentucky. Part of her current research is devoted to issues related to African American males, caregivers and Black faculty at Predominantly White Institutions (PWIs). She co-edited the text *Dilemmas of Black Faculty at Predominantly White Institutions in the United States: Issues in the Post-Multicultural Era* (The Edwin Mellen Press). She was awarded the 8th Annual Florence W. Vigilante Award for Scholarly Excellence for the article she coauthored in the *Journal of Teaching in Social Work*, "The Dehumanization of Black Males by Police: Teaching Social Justice – Black Life Really Does Matter."

Chapter 13
Social Justice Implications for Black Men's Health: Policing Black Bodies

Michael A. Robinson

Introduction

Before the official documentation of slavery in the United States, the mistreatment of Black men can be traced back to 1619. From the time slavery began in the states in the 1770s until its abolishment in the late 1860s, the practices of slavery plagued the lives of Africans and African Americans. While the official term and practice of slavery became illegal after the Civil War in December of 1865, the fair treatment of African Americans and Black persons never progressed, especially towards Black or African American men. The mistreatment, racism, oppression, and disenfranchisement of Black people took the form of Jim Crow Laws, the Black Codes, and the war on drugs. Once again, these new practices and laws plagued the lives of many African Americans and Black individuals (Robinson, 2017).

While America has made social progress since the 1770s, the same concepts, laws, practices, and beliefs that were once legal are still practiced today in the form of *The New Jim Crow*, stop and frisk, the over-incarceration of Black males, and the over-policing of Black communities and Black male bodies. Therefore, social justice organizations, social movements, social workers, and public health workers highlight and fight against discriminatory and social injustice practices to create an equal society for all Americans.

M. A. Robinson (✉)
School of Social Work, University of Georgia, Athens, GA, USA
e-mail: marobi01@uga.edu

Top 10 Leading Causes of Death in Black Men

According to the Centers for Disease Control and Prevention (CDC), the top 10 leading causes of death of Black Non-Hispanic Males in 2017 are: (1) heart disease, (2) cancer, (3) unintentional injuries, (4) homicide, (5) stroke, (6) diabetes, (7) chronic lower respiratory diseases, (8) kidney disease, (9) septicemia, and (10) hypertension (Heron, 2019). From this list, we can see that homicide is among the top five leading causes of death among Black men. When broken down by age, the number one leading cause of death among Black males between the ages of 1–19 years (35.3%) and 20–44 years (27.6%) is homicide, which is the ninth leading cause of death for Black males between the ages of 45–64 years (2.1%) (Heron, 2019).

When comparing and examining the top 10 leading causes of death for White males overall, homicide is not in the top 10 for this particular group. However, homicide is the ninth leading cause of death for Hispanic males. When broken down by age, homicide is not a top leading cause of death for White Non-Hispanic males and Hispanic males. Homicide is ranked as the fourth leading cause of death for White males aged 1–19 years (5.2%) and the fifth leading cause of death for White males between the ages of 20–44 years (2.8%). For Hispanic males, homicide is the second leading cause of death for men aged 1–19 years (14.4%) and the third leading cause of death for those aged 20–44 years (10.6%) (Heron, 2019). Figure 13.1 reflects the rate of homicide deaths when broken down by age and race. While the data shows that the rate of homicide decreases with age, Black males still have an overall higher rate of homicide deaths when compared to their White and Hispanic counterparts. Although the events or individuals involved in the rates of homicide,

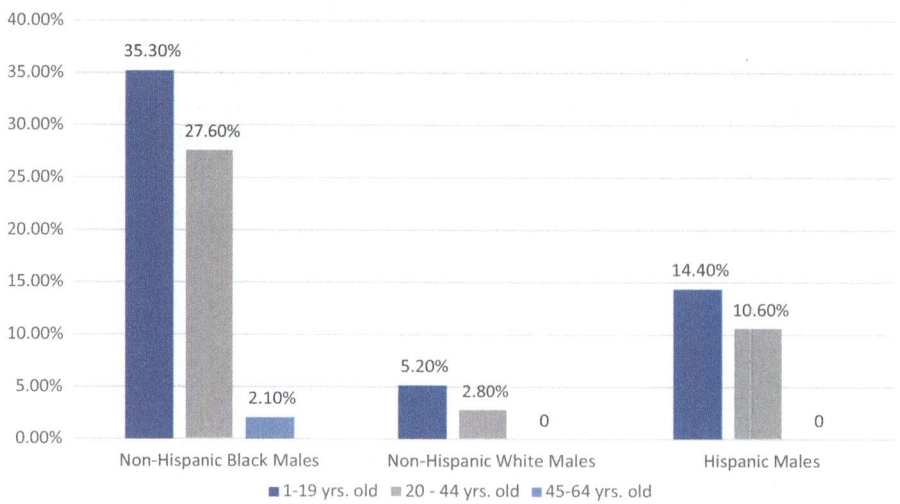

Fig. 13.1 Rate of male homicides broken down by age and race

it is important to note that homicide does not only focus on homicide committed by civilians. Homicides also include deaths caused by police and law enforcement.

Police Violence Against Black Men as a Public Health Concern

To understand how police violence is a health concern, it is essential to conceptualize police violence and public health concern. According to Moore (2020), police violence and/or brutality is the use of illegal excessive and unjustified force against community members, resulting in individuals feeling higher forms of distress, requiring medical attention, or death. Police violence and brutality range from but are not limited to assault, battery, torture, harassment, intimidation, mistreatment, verbal abuse, and murder. According to the CDC Foundation (n.d.), public health is the pursuit, understanding, and application of how public health professionals can protect and improve people's overall health and quality of life, neighborhoods, communities, and countries. According to Young et al. (2018), examples of public health concerns are alcohol-related harms, food safety, healthcare-associated infections, heart disease and stroke, and HIV. These public health concerns are addressed to reduce and eventually prevent these concerns from occurring at higher rates. To accomplish this goal, public health professionals partner with other professionals across different disciplines to identify and implement educational programs, examine and advocate for policy changes, provide community services and resources, and conduct research (CDC Foundation, n.d.).

Due to the adverse health consequences of police and law enforcement involvement, the American Public Health Association (APHA) (2018) recognized law enforcement violence as a public health issue because of the rates of disproportionality of law enforcement interaction minority groups were facing, primarily Black and African American males. With increased interactions with police or law enforcement, Black males are more likely to experience higher economic costs, psychological violence, and physical violence, which are fundamental concepts that impact public health.

Each year, over 200 million Americans are stopped by police and law enforcement officers due to traffic violations. As a result, this is the most common form of interaction Americans have with law enforcement (Langton & Durose, 2013; Pierson et al., 2020). Philando Castile had a history of being stopped by police. Castile was stopped at least 46 times in 14 years for impeding traffic, not wearing a seat belt, failure to slow down, and running a stop sign. Abrahams (2020) highlights "two main conjectures: 1) almost everyone on the road is committing some form of minor infraction for which an officer could pull them over, and 2) when someone is repeatedly stopped for minor infractions, the real reason may be something other than what is written on his traffic tickets" (p. 1). Similar to Philando Castile who was driving who was driving while Black, being racial profiled is a reality that many Black Americans face everyday. Consequently, the potential for a negative outcome significantly increases for Black individuals, especially Black males.

Utilizing the FBI arrest and NVSS injury data, Miller et al. (2017) highlighted how Black individuals experience higher rates of arrest/stop rates in addition to higher rates of legal intervention deaths when compared to White individuals. Between 1999 and 2013, deaths due to legal intervention increased by 45% (0.11 to 0.16/100,000) with higher rates among Black individuals (0.24) when compared to "American Indian/Alaska Natives (0.20); and Hispanic Whites (0.17) compared with non-Hispanic whites (0.09) and Asian/Pacific Islanders (0.05)" (DeGue et al., 2016, p. S174), represented in Fig. 13.2. Moreover, Black males experience higher victimization rates as a direct result of law enforcement intervention.

Krieger et al. (2015) examined trends in the United States due to legal intervention among Black and White men. Between 1960 and 2010, 15,699 deaths in the United States were due to legal intervention. Of these deaths, 55.3% (5489) were White men, and 42.3% (4204) were Black men. While White men had a higher rate of death, the death rate of Black men due to law enforcement intervention was 3–4 times higher than that of the US Black population "(e.g., 1960: 10.5% black, 88.6% white; 2010: 12.6% black, 72.4% white)" (Krieger et al., 2015, p. 2). More current research presented by Edwards, Lee, and Esposito (2019) highlights the risk of being killed by police in the United States by age, race, and sex. Between 2013 and 2018, roughly 1 in every 1000 Black men can expect to be killed by police over a life course. Moreover, Black men are 2.5 times more likely to be killed by police than their White male counterparts. It has also been noted that police kill Black men between 25 and 29 years of age at a higher rate than any other race (2.8 and 4.1 per 100,000) throughout the life course; White men 0.9 and 1.4 per 100,000; Latino men 1.4 and 2.2 per 100,000; and American Indian and Alaska Native men 1.5 and 2.8 per 100,000. While police use of force deaths account for 0.05% of all males' deaths

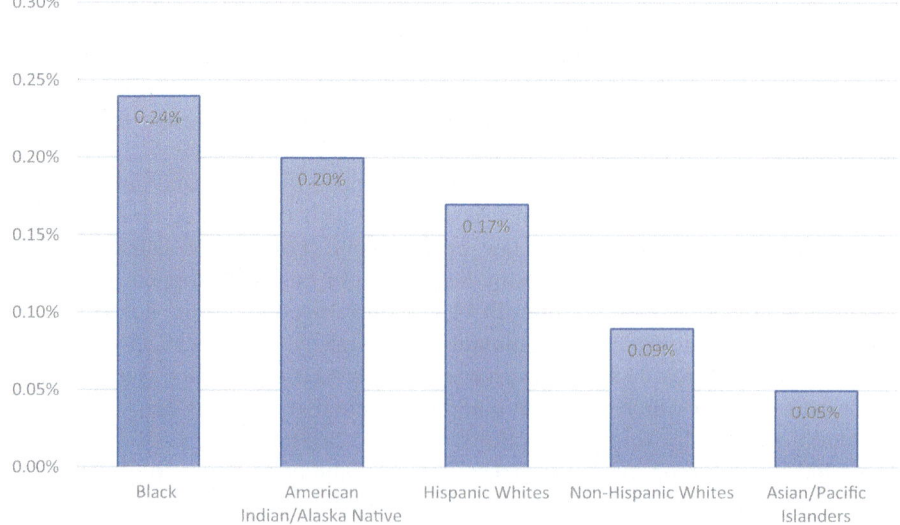

Fig. 13.2 Deaths due to legal intervention between 1999 and 2013

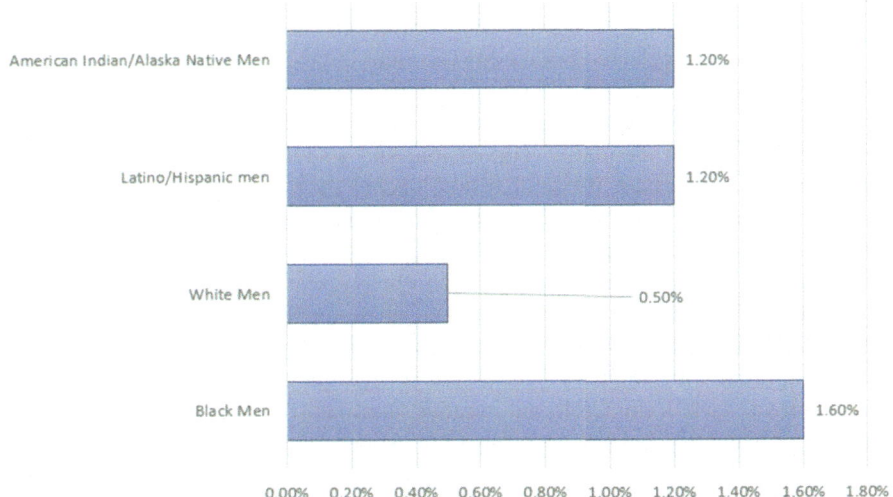

Fig. 13.3 Rate of deaths of men between the ages of 20–24 years by police. (Source: Edwards et al., 2019)

in the United States, the disproportionality between racial groups is consistent with other trends and research. Highlighted in Fig. 13.3, Edwards et al., (2019) show how law enforcement intervention was responsible for 1.6% of deaths of Black males between 20 and 24 years old, which is higher than that of White (0.5%), Latino (1.2%), and American Indian/Alaska Native (1.2%) males in the same age range.

Research and studies have highlighted the disproportionality of law enforcement intervention resulting in the violence and death of Black men as a result of their race (Adedoyin et al., 2018; Moore et al., 2017). While race and racism are key factors in predicting individuals' health outcomes, society must understand how race plays a role in the complexities of structural racism, in turn affecting the overall public health of Black males.

Theoritical Framework

The most prominent theory to help understand and change why and how race plays a role in the violence and killing of Black men at the hands of police is the Critical Race Theory (CRT). The Critical Race Theory initially emerged as a law movement during the Civil Rights era and was derived from Critical Legal Studies (CLS). Critical Legal Studies highlighted how "the law tends to enforce, reflect, constitute, and legitimize the dominant social and power relations through social actors who generally believe that they are neutral and arrive at their decisions through an objective process of legal reasoning…American Law and legal institutions tend to serve and to legitimize an oppressive social order" (Brown & Jackson, 2013, p. 12). While the CLS provided perceptiveness into the workings of the legal system and process, the CLS movement neglected to take into account the experiences and struggles of minorities, people of color, specifically Black people (Brown & Jackson, 2013). As a result of the CLS not accounting for Black experiences, the CRT offers a historical context of how racial inequality, oppression, and social injustices are present in today's society. Moreover, it captures how deeply race is ingrained in American society's institutional structure, elucidating how violence towards and killing Black men is an inescapable reality as it was in the past (Adedoyin et al., 2019).

Theories are conceptualized and framed to help researchers and scholars understand and explain behaviors, challenges, and phenomena. However, Critical Race Theory (CRT) is an iterative methodological practice in which it applies an action-oriented approach to improve processes, procedures, and problems (Ford & Airhihenbuwa, 2010). In CRT, an iterative approach encourages scholars and researchers to identify and stay attentive to injustices to transform systems that perpetuate any cycles of racial inequalities discovered throughout their research (Ford & Airhihenbuwa, 2010). Therefore, CRT can incorporate and adopt transdisciplinary methodologies, experienced-based knowledge, and critical knowledge to bring greater attention and awareness to combat the root causes of institutionalized and structural racism (Ford & Airhihenbuwa, 2010).

One core concept and tenet of CRT is how deeply racism is structurally engrained and built into US systems, institutions, and cultures but is not recognized (Adedoyin et al., 2019; Siegel, 2020). Law enforcement agencies are institutions where racism is deeply ingrained into their laws, systems, and policies. As a result, minorities, especially Black males, are mistreated and face unjust consequences, keeping them in a position of oppression and powerlessness. Thus, the CRT illustrates how violence and killing of Black males by police are an inescapable, persistent, and consistent reality. However, within institutions such as law enforcement agencies where racism is ingrained other forms of racism have been identified by integrating the Critical Race Theory into a public health model (Jones, 2000; Siegel, 2020). One form of racism is personally mediated racism. Personally mediated racism is described as being the most common and notable form of racism. It highlights prejudices, discriminatory acts, and biases against another individual. The next form is institutionalized racism. This form of racism illuminates unequal access to rights, privileges, resources, and powers facilitated by societal structures and institutions. The last form of racism derived from the Critical Race Theory and public health model is personalized racism. Personalized racism is the mental and psychological effects of labeling, stigmatization, and persecution of minorities, especially Black males (Jones, 2000).

Providing a historical context to present-day racial injustices, inequalities, and oppression, the Critical Race Theory challenges the traditional and conventional way of thinking about racism, how it can be eliminated and how racial inequality and oppression should be analyzed. While recognizing racism is a part of the Critical Race Theory, it is important to note that personally mediated, institutionalized, and personalized racism would not eliminate racism from occurring. From a Critical

Race Theory perspective, racism cannot only be viewed as an unjust process; it must also be considered as unmerited and discriminatory consequences for those who are discriminated against. Thusly, the liberation of Black males from police brutality and violence cannot occur without addressing the history of enslavement, past and present-day discrimination and inequality, and present life disadvantages (Adedoyin et al., 2019, Siegel, 2020; Jones, 2000).

Social Justice Implications

Since its origin in 2013, Black Lives Matter has sought and fought for social justice and policy change in the United States. In 2020, George Floyd was handcuffed and killed by the hands of a White police officer kneeling on his neck for approximately 9 min and 30 s. During this time, George Floyd screamed that he could not breathe. Despite his plea for air and being recorded, the White officer refused to take his knee off Floyd's neck, resulting in his death. As a result of his death, Black Lives Matter social movements sparked across the world. While these social movements are essential and vital for change, social justice implications cannot occur without the cooperation of federal, state/local level agencies, and civilian/community level members.

Social justice implications at the federal level should include congress allocating and increasing funds to the Department of Justice (DOJ) for Section 14141. Section 1414 is under the Violent Crime Act of 1994, which grants the DOJ the legal authority to launch an investigation and pursue legal action against law enforcement agencies deemed to have engaged in a systemic violation of constitutional or statutory law (Carter, 2016, Chanin, 2016). By hiring more investigators to enforce Section 1414, law enforcement agencies are more inclined to monitor officers' actions and modify departmental policy standards to avoid formal legal action (Carter, 2016). Another federal implication noted by Carter (2016) is updating reporting standards and following recommendations outlined in "The President's Task Force on 21st Century Policing," signed by former president Barack Obama after the Ferguson protest. The task force highlights six pillars of policing that are needed to rebuild community relations. If the DOJ requires law enforcement agencies to follow strict reporting policies, the DOJ can analyze data to ensure it falls in line with the six pillars. As a result, it will force the DOJ to hold law enforcement agencies accountable, requiring them to modify their policing behaviors to ensure compliance.

Implications at the state and local level should focus on revising and enhancing law enforcement curricula, including sensitivity training, cultural biases training, and protecting human rights (Moore et al., 2016; Carter, 2016) to combat social injustices that are demonstrated by law enforcement personnel. Enhancing law enforcement curricula can lead to intentional actions to reform law enforcement practices and agencies through a social justice lens. However, for this implication to be effective, law enforcement curricula need to emphasize continuing education units (CEU). Similar to other professions where continuing education units are required, the same requirement should be mandatory for law enforcement. Implementing the strategy of enchaining policing curricula can lead to officers recognizing racial and other biases, bringing about a sense of self-awareness, and finally, better practices for policing strategies and approaches when interacting with Black and African American individuals (Moore et al., 2016).

Another state- and/or local-level implication that could make a difference and combat social injustice is law enforcement agencies making an effort to recruit and hire more people of color (POC) or people that reflect the communities they serve (Carter, 2016). Hiring officers that reflect the community in which they serve can have a positive impact. For example, it can help rebuild the police-citizen relationship, reduce racial tensions and biases, and provide a community's historical and structural background. Moreover, these officers will have more knowledge and empathy toward cultural sensitivities, thusly increasing problem-solving and innovative policing strategies for interacting with minority communities and individuals (Theobald & Haider-Markel, 2009; Carter, 2016; Fifield, 2016, Legewie, & Fagan, 2016). Moreover, hiring more POC officers can reduce the stigma officers face from minority communities and dismantle racial solidarity within predominately White law enforcement agencies. When law enforcement agencies lack diversity, there is an increase in group situational thinking in addition to greater shared values, beliefs, increasing police unity, increasing the "us" vs. "them" mentality (Fifield, 2016; Portes, & Sensenbrenner, 1993; Legewie, & Fagan, 2016).

At the civilian or community level, community leaders should engage in proactive intervention strategies (Moore et al., 2016). Community leaders hold a social power within the community that can ignite change. Community leaders, constructing programs or events that allow for partnerships with law enforcement agencies, can help rebuild the community–police relationship, especially among Black and African American youth. Furthermore, it will create a safe space for community members and police, allowing for opportunities to break down racial stigmas and biases, encourage in-depth conversations, and increase police-community interactions positively. As a result, connections within the community can begin to thrive, allowing community leaders and police to brainstorm solutions for more effective policing.

Conclusion

Throughout history, we have witnessed and documented the mistreatment against Black and African American individuals, especially Black males. However, the disregard and dismissal of police violence and the death of Black men by predominately White police and law enforcement officers show history is repeating itself in a different form. As a result, police violence against Black individuals has been identified as a public health concern by public health professionals. To combat the disproportionality of deaths and violence by police, institutions have to understand the historical context and background of race in our country and how it is woven into society's structures and systems. From the Civil Rights Movement to the Black Lives Matter social movement, the fight for social justice and equality had been a battle for 70 years for a Black individual. While social justice implications and police reform are gaining momentum due to social movements, state and federal level agencies have to take the initiative, address these injustices, enforce policy changes, and hold officers and agencies accountable for their actions. Until the first step toward change begins, the death trends of Black men at the hands of law enforcement officers will not only reflect past and current research but also have the potential to increase, resulting in the death of more Black men.

Summary

This chapter focuses on the killing of African American men by police and how it has become a public health crisis. The most prominent theory to help understand and change why and how race plays a role in the violence and killing of Black men at the hands of police is Critical Race Theory. Last, the author introduces and discusses social justice implications for policy changes at the federal, state, and local levels.

Discussion Questions

1. Describe in detail how police violence against Black men is considered a public health crisis.
2. How does Critical Race Theory explain and predict police violence and discriminatory practices by law enforcement in the Black community?
3. What has prompted social justice movements like "Black Lives Matter" to erupt worldwide? Has the movement made a difference? If yes, how so? And if no, why not?
4. More White men have been killed by police than Black men, so why is it that deaths of Black men are considered a public health crisis?

Exercises

1. Compare and contrast the tenets of Critical Race Theory (CRT) and the Black Lives Matter Movement.
2. Use the Tenets of CRT to explain to your classmates why police killings of unarmed Black men are a public health crisis.
3. What suggestions or strategies do you have for public health officials for addressing the crisis of police killings of unarmed Black men?
4. How would you address a graduating class from the police academy that is being assigned to work in the Black community? What suggestions might you have?

Glossary of Terms and Concepts

Black Codes: These were very restrictive laws/customs enacted after the official end of slavery. They were designed to keep the newly freed slaves in the south to provide cheap labor.

Critical Race Theory: A theory or movement developed by Kimberlé Crenshaw that forces a critical look at race and racism across society and how race really matters in America.

Jim Crow: Named after a fictional character, these were customs that were enacted after Reconstruction in the south. These customs maintained a system of segregation that lasted from the late 1800s through the Civil Rights Movement of the 1960s.

Personally Mediated Racism: It is defined as prejudice and discrimination, where prejudice means differential assumptions about the abilities, motives, and intentions of others according to their race and discrimination means differential actions toward others according to their race (Jones, 2000).

New Jim Crow: A 2010 text by Michelle Alexander where she writes about her belief that mass incarceration in the era of colorblindness is the rebirth of Jim Crow.

Stop and Frisk: A tactic enacted by police departments to stop and detain suspected criminals for no legal reason except to look for contraband such as drugs or illegal firearms.

War on Drugs: This is a movement that started in the 1970s that was an initiative designed to stop the illegal drug trade by increasing prison terms drastically for drug dealers and users. This initiative is still in effect today

References

Abrahams, S. (2020). Officer differences in traffic stops of minority drivers. *Labour Economics, 67*, 101912.

Adedoyin, C., Robinson, M., Clayton, D. M., Moore, S., Jones-Eversley, S., Crosby, S., & Boamah, D. A. (2018). A synergy of contemporary activism to address police maltreatment of black males: An intersectional analysis. *Journal of Human Behavior in the Social Environment, 28*(8), 1078–1090.

Adedoyin, A. C., Moore, S. E., Robinson, M. A., Clayton, D. M., Boamah, D. A., & Harmon, D. K. (2019). The dehumanization of black males by police: Teaching social justice—Black life really does matter! *Journal of Teaching in Social Work, 39*(2), 111–131.

American Public Health Association. (2018). *Addressing law enforcement violence as a public health issue*. American Public Health Association. Retrieved March 6, 2021, from https://www.apha.org/policies-and-advocacy/public-health-policy-statements/policy-database/2019/01/29/law-enforcement-violence

Brown, K., & Jackson, D. D. (2013). The history and conceptual elements of critical race theory. In *Handbook of critical race theory in education* (pp. 9–22). Routledge.

Carter, C. A. (2016). Police brutality, the law & today's social justice movement: How the lack of police accountability has fueled# hashtag activism. *CUNY Law Review, 20*, 521.

CDC Foundation. (n.d.). *What is public health?* CDC Foundation. Retrieved March 6, 2021, from https://www.cdcfoundation.org/what-public-health

Chanin, J. (2016). Evaluating Section 14141: An empirical review of pattern or practice police misconduct reform. *Ohio State Journal of Criminal Law, 14*, 67.

DeGue, S., Fowler, K. A., & Calkins, C. (2016). Deaths due to use of lethal force by law enforcement: Findings from the national violent death reporting system, 17 U.S. states, 2009–2012. *American journal of preventive medicine, 51*(5), S173–S187.

Edwards, F., Lee, H., & Esposito, M. (2019). Risk of being killed by police use of force in the United States by age, race–ethnicity, and sex. *Proceedings of the National Academy of Sciences, 116*(34), 16793–16798.

Fifield, J. (2016). Does diversifying police forces reduce tensions. *Pew Trusts*.

Ford, C. L., & Airhihenbuwa, C. O. (2010). Critical race theory, race equity, and public health: Toward antiracism praxis. *American Journal of Public Health, 100*(S1), S30–S35.

Heron, M. P. (2019). *Deaths: Leading causes for 2017*.

Jones, C. P. (2000). Levels of racism: a theoretic framework and a gardener's tale. *American Journal of Public Health, 90*(8), 1212.

Krieger, N., Kiang, M. V., Chen, J. T., & Waterman, P. D. (2015). Trends in U.S. deaths due to legal intervention among black and white men, age 15–34 years, by county income level. *Harvard Public Health Review, 3*, 1–5.

Langton, L., & Durose, M. (2013). *Police behavior during traffic and street stops, 2011* (Technical report). U.S. Department of Justice.

Legewie, J., & Fagan, J. (2016). Group threat, police officer diversity and the deadly use of police force. *Columbia Public Law Research Paper* (14-512).

Miller, T. R., Lawrence, B. A., Carlson, N. N., Hendrie, D., Randall, S., Rockett, I. R., & Spicer, R. S. (2017). Perils of police action: A cautionary tale from US data sets. *Injury Prevention: Journal of the International Society for Child and Adolescent Injury Prevention, 23*(1), 27–32. https://doi.org/10.1136/injuryprev-2016-042023

Moore, L. (2020, July 27). Police brutality in the United States. In *Encyclopedia britannica*.

Moore, S. E., Robinson, M. A., Adedoyin, A. C., Brooks, M., Harmon, D. K., & Boamah, D. (2016). Hands up—Don't shoot: Police shooting of young Black males: Implications for social work and human services. *Journal of Human Behavior in the Social Environment, 26*(3–4), 254–266.

Moore, S. E., Adedoyin, A. C., Brooks, M., Robinson, M. A., Harmon, D. K., & Boamah, D. A. (2017). Black Males living in an antithetical police culture: Keys for their survival. *Journal of Aggression, Maltreatment & Trauma, 26*(8), 902–919.

Pierson, E., Simoiu, C., Overgoor, J., Corbett-Davies, S., Jenson, D., Shoemaker, A., … Goel, S. (2020). A large-scale analysis of racial disparities in police stops across the United States. *Nature Human Behaviour, 4*(7), 736–745.

Portes, A., & Sensenbrenner, J. (1993). Embeddedness and immigration: Notes on the social determinants of economic action. *American Journal of Sociology, 98*(6), 1320–1350.

Robinson, M. A. (2017). Black bodies on the ground: Policing disparities in the African American community—An analysis of newsprint from January 1, 2015, through December 31, 2015. *Journal of Black Studies, 48*(6), 551–571. https://doi.org/10.1177/0021934717702134

Siegel, M. (2020). Racial disparities in fatal police shootings: An empirical analysis informed by critical race theory. *BUL Review, 100*, 1069.

Theobald, N. A., & Haider-Markel, D. P. (2009). Race, bureaucracy, and symbolic representation: Interactions between citizens and police. *Journal of Public Administration Research and Theory, 19*(2), 409–426.

Young, A. C., Lowry, G., Mumford, K., & Graaf, C. (2018). CDC's prevention status reports: Monitoring the status of public health policies and practices for improved performance and accountability. *Journal of public health management and practice: JPHMP, 24*(2), 121.

Michael A. Robinson, PhD, received his MSSW and PhD from the Raymond A. Kent School of Social Work and Family Science at the University of Louisville. He is currently a professor at the University of Georgia School of Social Work, where he serves as the Director of MSW Admissions. Dr. Robinson also serves as a board member on the Council on Social Work Education (CSWE), where he also serves as the Chair of the Commission for Diversity and Social and Economic Justice. Dr. Robinson has written the 2017 award-winning article, "Black bodies on the ground: Policing disparities in the African American community: A content analysis of newsprint from January 1, 2015 thru December 31, 2015" and also co-authored the 2019 award-winning article, "The dehumanization of Black Males by Police: Teachings in Social Justice—Black Life Really Does Matter." Dr. Robinson is also co-author of the book, *Police Shooting of Unarmed Black Males: Advancing Novel Prevention and Intervention Strategies* (Routledge, 2018). Dr. Robinson continues to publish in the area of police violence against African American men.

Index

A

Adverse Childhood Experiences (ACEs), 93
African American men
   coronary heart disease (CHD), 18
   health disparities, 18
   mortality and life expectancy, 18
African-centered practice, 81
Afrocentric cultural strengths-based
   approach, 89
American Medical Association (AMA), 110
American Psychiatric Association (2013), 113
American Public Health Association
   (APHA), 171
Anti-racist, 59
Anxiety disorders, 32
Assessment, Review, Manage and Monitor
   (ARMM), 51

B

Biological malfunction, 62
Black abolitionists, 156
Black activism and Black social
   movements, 155
Black athletes
   African American, 160
   African American intellectuals, 158
   BLM, 162
   interracial competition, 157
   Olympic carriers, 159
   police brutality and racial injustice, 165
   police brutality/mass incarceration,
      160, 161
Black codes, 177

Black community, 37
Black disease, 18
Black emancipation activism, 155
Black feminism, 71
Black Lives Matter (BLM), 177
Black males, 47, 50, 51, 53
Black masculinity, 60, 64
   cisgender, patriarchal and dominant, 73
   complicit form, 70
   dominant/hegemonic form, 70
   and intersectionality, 71
   marginalization, 70
   as "masculinities", 82
   remixing, 80
   and social movements, 72–73
   social science research and practice, 74
   subordinate form, 70
Black men
   at-risk, 70
   Civil Rights movement, 72
   fight to stop the killing, 73
   grounding behavior, 71
   intellectual and social framing, 72
   in leadership, 73
   masculinity, 70
   races and ethnicities, 71 Social justice
      implications
   "remix", 74
   victims of oppression, 72
Black men, culture
   African American Men, 91
   African drums, 85
   communities, 91
   culture strength, 88

Black men, culture (*cont.*)
   group development, 92
   men healing men and communities, 89–91
   MHMCN, 94, 95
   personal identity development, 93
   professional development, 93, 94
   rites of passages, 86, 87
   ROPE curriculum, 92
   social workers, 95, 96
   strengths-based approach, 86, 87
   values/practices, 88
   violence and trauma, 91
Black men's health destabilization, 7
Black mental health
   American communities, 30
   anxiety disorders, 30
   cancer diagnosis, 29
   community, 29
   cultural humility, 40
   depression, 30
   discrimination, 31
   disparities, 38
   distrust of healthcare, 31–33
   double consciousness, 40
   government response to crisis, 31–33
   health outcomes, 29
   interpersonal barriers
      African American, 33
      behavior, 33
      challenges, 33
      cultural humility, 33–35
      decentralization of whiteness, 33–35
      implication, 33
      invisibility to transformation, 35, 36
   mental disorders, 30
   post-traumatic stressors, 30
   racial group, 29
   racism, 31
   somebodiness, 41
   transformative action, 29
   trauma, 30
   United States, 30, 38
   whiteness, 40
Black, Indigenous, and People of Color
      (BIPOC), 62, 63, 142
BLM movement, 109

C
Capabilities Approach, 37, 38
Capitalism, 59, 60, 62
Centers for Disease Control and Prevention
      (CDC), 110, 121

Chronic Disease Self-Management Program
      (CDSMP), 22, 23
Civil rights activists, 164
Civil Rights Movement, 177
Civil War, 31
Cleveland Summit, 164
Clinical Social Work's Contribution to a Social
      Justice Perspective, 115
Colonialism, 58, 60
Collaboration, 102, 103
Colonial logic, 59
Colonial modes of disqualification, 61
Colonization, 58, 60, 61
Colonized, 60, 61
Colonizer, 60, 61, 63
Communities Partnership for Peace Initiative
      (CP4P), 79
Community-Based Organization (CBO), 106
Congress on Racial Equality (CORE),
      102, 158
Co-productive methodologies, 35
Counter-storytelling, 143
COVID-19 pandemic, 31, 95, 140
   infections, 7
   testing and vaccinations, 95
Critical Legal Studies (CLS), 173, 174
Critical psychology, 64
Critical race studies (CRS), 142
Critical race theory (CRT), 36, 37, 40, 71, 142,
      146, 156, 173, 174, 177
Cultural competence, 34
Cultural phenomenon, 32
Cure Violence, 79

D
Department of Justice (DOJ), 175
Depression, 111
Diagnostic and Statistical Manual of Mental
      Disorders (DSM), 35
Diagnostic and Statistical Manual of Mental
      Disorders, Fifth Edition
      (DSM-5), 117
Discourse, 58, 59
Double consciousness, 40
Driving While Black (DWB), 111

F
Faith and spirituality, 8–9
Fascist modes
   of social organization, 59
Faulty neurology, 62

Filer Commission, 102
Food and Drug Administration (FDA), 121

G
Gender-influenced stereotypes, 137
Genocide, 32
Gun Violence Intervention and Prevention, 94

H
Health and Recovery Peer (HARP), 22
Healthcare, 48
Healthcare systems
   AIDS, 135
   American healthcare systems, 136
   Black men's health, 136, 138
   CRS, 142, 143
   CRT, African American/Black men, 144
   engagement framework, 146, 147
   finances/economic stability, 137
   gender-influenced stereotypes, 137
   health disparities, 136, 138
   health equity, 136
   incarceration, 139, 140
   medicine, black male representation, 140, 141
   personal health management, 139
   racism/mistrust, 136, 137
   religion/faith-based ideology, 138
   social determinants, 136
Health-related quality of life (HRQOL), 22
Healthy lifestyle, 17
Historical and structural racism, 145
Historical collective trauma, 62
Historical narratives, 75
Human Capital Initiative, 122
Human suffering, 61, 62
Hyper-policing, 7

I
Innovative strategies
   activities, 128
   barriers, 121–123
   engaging, 122, 123, 125
   government-funded activities, 121
   innovative and best practices, 123, 124
   research, 121–123
   stress, 121
Innovative Tailored-Recruitment Interventions
      (iTRI), 123, 125, 126, 129
Integrated health services, 106
Intentional tailored-research techniques (ITT),
      123–125, 129

Internal Revenue Code, 102
Internal Revenue Service (IRS), 102
Intersectionality, 40, 71, 73, 74
Intersectionality theory, 116, 117
Intersectional theory, 144
IQ tests, 62, 63

J
Jim Crow, 178

L
Law enforcement, 171, 173, 175, 177
Legalized chattel system, 156
Liberation psychology, 64
Licensed Clinical Social Worker (LCSW), 51
Lung cancer, 135

M
Mainstream psychology, 62
Masculinity
   complicit form, 70
   dominant/hegemonic form, 70
   hegemonic masculinity, 72
   intersectionality, 71
   marginalization, 70
   social construct, 70
   social descriptor, 70
   social movements and Black
      masculinity, 72–73
   subordinate form, 70
Masking strategy, 75
Master signifier, 58–60
Men Healing Men and Communities
      (MHMCN), 89
Men of Color Health Awareness (MOCHA),
      123, 126, 127
Mental health, 51, 58–61
Mental health effects, 111
Metropolitan Peace Academy (MPA), 79, 80

N
Narrative therapy, 64
National Academies of Sciences, 109
National Alliance on Mental Health
      (NAMI), 88
National Association for the Advancement of
      Colored People (NAACP), 102, 158
National Association of Social Workers
      (NASW), 115
National Institutes of Health (NIH), 121

National Survey of children, 48
New Jim Crow, 169, 178
Nonprofit Charitable Organization, 106
Nonprofit organizations, 103
Nonprofit Social Welfare Organization, 107

O
Office of Minority Health, 104, 105
Olympic Project for Human Rights (OPHR), 159

P
People of color (POC), 176
Personal health management, 139
Personalized innovative comprehensive (PIC),
        123, 126, 129
Personally mediated racism, 178
Police brutality, 109, 111, 113, 114
Police violence, 171–173
Positive Youth Development (PYD), 48–50, 53
Post-exposure prophylaxis (PrEP), 144
Prisoner reentry industry (PRI), 6
Prison industrial complex (PIC), 6
Psychosocial factors, 114
Psychosocial oppression, 8
Psychotherapy, 61
Psychotic fantasy, 61
Puberty rites, 74

R
Racial bias, 69
Racial discrimination, 51
Racial trauma
        depression, 112
        microaggressions, 112, 113
        racial discrimination, 112
Racism, 58, 59, 62
Radical social work, 64
Reflexivity, 115
Remix, 69, 74, 80, 82
Respectability politics, 73
Rites, 74
Rites of passage (ROP) program, 74–76
Rites of passages experience (ROPE), 92
Robert Wood Johnson Foundation, 34

S
Schizophrenia, 31
Self-management
        cardiac rehabilitation (CR), 21
        disease management program, 21
        HARP, 22

health diagnosis, 19
        Healthy Together program, 23, 24
        HRQOL, 22
        programs, 20
        self-efficacy, 19
        serious mental illness (SMI), 22
        Spanish-speaking patients, 20
        Women Take PRIDE program, 21
Service delivery system
        black community, 104
        community-based nonprofit
                organizations, 106
        community-based resources, 101
        complexity, 101
        healthcare, 101
        inequalities, 101
        inequities, 101
        inequity gap, 106
        integrated healthcare, 105
        nonprofit organizations, 102
        organizations, 102
        service integration, 102–104
        social and economic support services, 104
Service integration, 102–104
Settler-colonial capitalism, 59
Signifier, 58
Social capital theory, 4
        bonding, 4
        bridging, 4
        concepts of, 4
        linking, 5
        structural and cognitive, 5
Social determinants of health (SDoH), 6
Social discourse, 59
Social inequities, 32
Social justice implications
        BLM, 175
        causes of death, 170, 171
        civilian/community level, 176
        community, 176
        human rights, 175
        law enforcement, 175
        legal, 169
        police violence, 171–173, 176
        public health concern, 171–173
        United States, 169
Social movements, 72–74
Social networking sites (SNS), 114
Social service intervention, 77
Social services, 72, 74
Social Work and Public Health, 9–11
Social workers, 115
Sociological theory, 116
Southern Christian Leadership Conference
        (SCLC), 102

Spatial justice, 37, 41
Spirituality, 75
State of Play, 48
Statistical tools, 63
Stop and frisk, 169, 178
Strength-based perspective, 57, 63, 87
Structural racism, 62, 63
Student Nonviolent Coordinating Committee
        (SNCC), 102, 158
Subaltern, 61
Subjectification, 59
Subjectivity, 58, 59
Systemic racism, 69

T
Toxic masculinity, 70
Traditional innovative customary (TIC), 123, 129
Trauma
    Black men, 109
    digital media and racism, 114
    high-profile cases, 109
    intersectionality theory, 116–118
    microaggressions, 118
    phenomenological experience, 118
    police violence, 109
    practice and treatment, 114, 115
    race, 110
    racial discrimination, 110, 117, 118
    racial trauma, 118
    racism, 110
    reflexivity, 119
    self-care, 118
    vicarious trauma, 119

Trauma training, 76
Truth n' Trauma Program (TNT), 76

U
Unontologize/ontology, 58

V
Violence impacts, 51

W
War on drugs, 169, 178
Whiteness, 40
World Health Organization (2001), 29

Y
Youth sports
    adulthood, 53
    ARMM, 51, 52
    Black youth, 50, 51
    challenges, 47, 53
    COVID pandemic, 48
    demographics, 48
    evidence-based research, 53
    literature, 53
    longitudinal studies, 53
    mental illness, 47
    PYD, 48–50
    social workers, 53
    team sports, 47
    trauma, 47

The manufacturer's authorised representative in the EU is Springer
Nature Customer Service Centre GmbH, Europaplatz 3, 69115 Heidelberg,
Germany. If you have any concerns regarding our products, please
contact ProductSafety@springernature.com

Printed and bound by CPI Group (UK) Ltd, Croydon, CR0 4YY
24/04/2026
02096317-0003